Focus on Family Historians:
How Ancestor Research Affects Self-Understanding and Well-Being

Focus on Family Historians: How Ancestor Research Affects Self-Understanding and Well-Being

Editors

Susan M Moore
Doreen Rosenthal

MDPI • Basel • Beijing • Wuhan • Barcelona • Belgrade • Manchester • Tokyo • Cluj • Tianjin

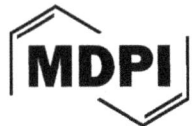

Editors
Susan M Moore
Faculty of Health, Arts and Design, Swinburne University of Technology,
P.O. Box 218,
Hawthorn, VIC 3122,
Australia

Doreen Rosenthal
Melbourne School of Population and Global Health, The University of Melbourne,
Victoria 3010, Australia

Editorial Office
MDPI
St. Alban-Anlage 66
4052 Basel, Switzerland

This is a reprint of articles from the Special Issue published online in the open access journal *Genealogy* (ISSN 2313-5778) (available at: https://www.mdpi.com/journal/genealogy/special_issues/Family_Historians).

For citation purposes, cite each article independently as indicated on the article page online and as indicated below:

LastName, A.A.; LastName, B.B.; LastName, C.C. Article Title. *Journal Name* **Year**, *Volume Number*, Page Range.

ISBN 978-3-0365-4149-5 (Hbk)
ISBN 978-3-0365-4150-1 (PDF)

Cover image courtesy of Susan Moore.

© 2022 by the authors. Articles in this book are Open Access and distributed under the Creative Commons Attribution (CC BY) license, which allows users to download, copy and build upon published articles, as long as the author and publisher are properly credited, which ensures maximum dissemination and a wider impact of our publications.
The book as a whole is distributed by MDPI under the terms and conditions of the Creative Commons license CC BY-NC-ND.

Contents

About the Editors vii

Susan M. Moore
How Ancestor Research Affects Self-Understanding and Well-Being: Introduction to the Special Issue
Reprinted from: *Genealogy* **2022**, *6*, 20, doi:10.3390/genealogy6010020 1

Antonia Bifulco
Family History and Searching for Hidden Trauma—A Personal Commentary
Reprinted from: *Genealogy* **2021**, *5*, 46, doi:10.3390/genealogy5020046 7

Graeme Aplin
Context: The Role of Place and Heritage in Genealogy
Reprinted from: *Genealogy* **2021**, *5*, 58, doi:10.3390/genealogy5020058 21

Susan M. Moore and Doreen A. Rosenthal
What Motivates Family Historians? A Pilot Scale to Measure Psychosocial Drivers of Research into Personal Ancestry
Reprinted from: *Genealogy* **2021**, *5*, 83, doi:10.3390/genealogy5030083 31

Rebecca Robinson
Pilgrimage and Purpose: Ancestor Research as Sacred Practice in a Secular Age
Reprinted from: *Genealogy* **2021**, *5*, 90, doi:10.3390/genealogy5040090 45

Emma L. Shaw and Debra J. Donnelly
(Re)discovering the Familial Past and Its Impact on Historical Consciousness
Reprinted from: *Genealogy* **2021**, *5*, 102, doi:10.3390/genealogy5040102 57

Gary Clapton
Family Histories, Family Stories and Family Secrets: Late Discoveries of Being Adopted
Reprinted from: *Genealogy* **2021**, *5*, 105, doi:10.3390/genealogy5040105 73

Pam Jarvis
Ancestral Selfies and Historical Traumas: Who Do You Feel You Are?
Reprinted from: *Genealogy* **2022**, *6*, 1, doi:10.3390/genealogy6010001 81

Helen Parker-Drabble
How Key Psychological Theories Can Enrich Our Understanding of Our Ancestors and Help Improve Mental Health for Present and Future Generations: A Family Historian's Perspective
Reprinted from: *Genealogy* **2022**, *6*, 4, doi:10.3390/genealogy6010004 93

Catherine Agnes Theunissen
The Effects of DNA Test Results on Biological and Family Identities
Reprinted from: *Genealogy* **2022**, *6*, 17, doi:10.3390/genealogy6010017 115

Lindsey Büster
From Human Remains to Powerful Objects: Ancestor Research from a Deep-Time Perspective
Reprinted from: *Genealogy* **2022**, *6*, 23, doi:10.3390/genealogy6010023 131

Pam Jarvis
Book Review: The Psychology of Family History
Reprinted from: *Genealogy* **2021**, *5*, 39, doi:10.3390/genealogy5020039 143

About the Editors

Susan M Moore is a widely published developmental social psychologist whose major research interests encompass both the adolescent and senior life stages. She is an Emeritus Professor of Psychology at Swinburne University, a Fellow of the Australian Psychological Society, and an active family historian.

Doreen Rosenthal is a developmental social psychologist. Her research interests include ageing and sexual and reproductive health. She is a Fellow of the Academy of Social Sciences in Australia, and in 2003, she was made an Officer in the Order of Australia for her national and international research.

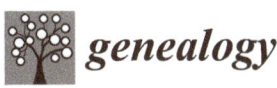

Editorial

How Ancestor Research Affects Self-Understanding and Well-Being: Introduction to the Special Issue

Susan M. Moore

Faculty of Health, Arts and Design, Swinburne University of Technology, Hawthorn, VIC 3122, Australia; smoore@swin.edu.au

Overview

The idea for this Special Issue of *Genealogy* came from my fascination not just with my own family history research, but through my involvement with groups of other passionate fellow family history researchers. As a retired psychological researcher, I was amazed at the intensity of emotions experienced by myself and others as we broke down research 'brick walls' and discovered more about our ancestors' lives. I was often moved to tears or laughter reading the stories that fellow family historians wrote on their blogs or Facebook pages, as well as being astounded at just how much enjoyable time could be spent indulging our hobby. In 2018, with Professor Emerita Doreen Rosenthal, my colleague and co-editor of this Special Issue, we conducted a survey of almost 1000 Australian hobbyist genealogists in part to answer the question, 'What motivates family historians?' We used the data collected, reviewed published literature, and took on board a fellow writer, Dr Rebecca Robinson, to produce the book, *The Psychology of Family History: Exploring our Genealogy*, published in 2021 by Taylor and Francis. Since we submitted our book for publication, not only has interest in family history increased greatly, so has curiosity about family historians! Research into the motives, outcomes and implications of discovering more about one's ancestors is expanding at a great rate. It seemed timely to capture some of this material in a Special Issue of *Genealogy* in which we 'Focus on Family Historians'.

Inviting scholars to contribute to the Special Issue, we sought articles that addressed several key topics, including explorations of the psychological and practical reasons people give for researching their family histories, the outcomes—both positive and negative—that ensue from the knowledge gained, and the notion that understanding one's ancestral background might promote personal growth and therapeutic change. A goal for the Special Issue was to foster a multi-disciplinary approach, so we sought research from sociology, psychology, history, family studies and other cognate disciplines, as well as encouraging a range of scholarly methodologies, including qualitative and quantitative empirical research, case material, literature reviews and discursive papers.

The ten articles (and one book review: (Jarvis 2021) presented here come from disciplines as varied as psychology/counselling, sociology, urban geography, theology, social work, communication studies, education and archaeology. Three general approaches are evident.

1. Scholarly interpretations of case-based material;
2. Empirical research;
3. Interpretive literature reviews.

1. Articles Based on Family History Case Material

Three authors (Bifulco 2021; Jarvis 2022; Parker-Drabble 2022) employed psychological theories to explain how events from their ancestral pasts such as forced migration, poverty and war can influence the personal and family narratives of current-day descendants. These narratives are the stories we tell ourselves—sometimes through feelings rather than words—about who we are and what constitutes our place in the world. They form part of

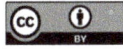

our identity or sense of self. As each of these authors acknowledges, Attachment Theory (e.g., Ainsworth and Bell 1970; Bowlby 1969, 1982) provides a model for explaining how trauma can move through the generations. Parenting is the key. A close, warm and loving relationship between infants and their caregivers, characterised by consistency of care, engenders a child's 'secure' attachment. This involves the child developing an understanding (based on their care) that the world is a trustworthy place and that their needs will be met. This kind of attachment is postulated as the basis for assured, confident adulthood and the ability to relate to others with warmth and integrity. However, some parenting styles promote insecure attachment, for example, caregivers who are highly anxious and self-doubting, or those who are neglectful, inconsistent or lacking in warmth. Historic trauma can engender insecure parenting. Mothers in concentration camps or families suffering the duress of extreme poverty may not be able to adequately attend to their babies. These children, if they survive, may be as damaged by the poverty of their early relationships as they were by the deprivation of their physical needs. In turn, they may experience problems in relating to their own offspring. In this way, as both Parker-Drabble and Bifulco demonstrate through case studies of their own families, insecure attachment can move through the generations with outcomes such as unresolved trauma, depression or addiction.

All three writers discuss the potential healing aspects of ancestral storytelling. Jarvis, using partially fictionalised family history scenarios, argues that when historical trauma becomes part of a family's narrative, descendants may be drawn to what Freud (1961) called 'traumatic re-enactment' through fantasy. This is a process that may be therapeutic or self-defeating. We may come to see ourselves as part of a long line of either victims or heroic survivors. Jarvis coins the lovely term 'historic selfie' to describe that aspect of a personal identity crafted through the 'psychic work' of incorporating ancestral stories into our sense of who we are.

Bifulco's paper, presenting her own ancestral story of wartime tragedy and trauma, notes the importance to the mental health of survivors (and their descendants) being able to talk about their experiences, give up their secrets and give vent to emotions like grief, sorrow, fear and guilt within a safe environment. Barriers to sharing the traumas of wartime include defensive forgetting, guilt and shame, but can also involve 'public forgetting' of unacknowledged national atrocities or failures. She writes: "When trauma is unresolved it can lead to many impacts including re-experiencing of the event and hypervigilance (e.g., through nightmares and flashbacks) but also avoidance of thinking about it (even amnesia for some events) as in PTSD. This can affect other family members such as children when it is witnessed in the domestic arena".

Parker-Drabble also stresses the therapeutic value gained from hearing (or discovering) ancestral stories. These can facilitate a deeper understanding of the forces that shaped the actions and personalities of our parents, grandparents and other key elders, thus paving the way for personal growth, for example through forgiveness, increased resilience or the motivation to change maladaptive coping styles.

The use of ancestral family history in mental health interventions, while acknowledged by some (e.g., Bhar and Silver 2016; Champagne 1990; Moore et al. 2021) is not yet widely practiced. Nevertheless, as Jarvis concludes, 'the concept of historical trauma is now well poised to move into mainstream psychology'.

2. Articles Based on Empirical Research

Three articles in the Special Issue report empirical studies of hobbyist family historians; one is survey-based and two focus on findings derived from in-depth interviews. The study by Shaw and Donnelly (2021) presents insights into historical thinking and research practices of four Australian family historians. Using the theoretical frameworks of Jorn Rüsen's Disciplinary Matrix (Rüsen 1993) and his Typology of Historical Consciousness (Rüsen 1996), these authors conclude that engaging in genealogical research shapes and refines researchers' historical understandings and consciousness. The study supports other findings that amateur family historians, even those with little or no historical training, are teaching themselves about the research methods of history and the nature of reliable evidence (e.g., Hershkovitz and Hardof-Jaffe 2017). In doing so, they are making important contributions to the history discipline and, as Shaw and Donnelly put it, "shifting the historical landscape through the dissemination of their research for public consumption beyond traditional family history audiences". In addition, through their new learnings and discoveries, these hobbyist genealogists experience personal growth through greater understanding of their place within a family context that extends backwards through history and is partly shaped by it.

An empirical study by the guest editors of this Special Issue (Moore and Rosenthal 2021) used quantitative and qualitative data from a large-scale survey of Australian amateur genealogical researchers to examine the motives that drive family historians to spend so much time, effort and passion on their hobby. Additionally, the data were used to develop a pilot form of a scale to measure these motives. Factor analysis of quantitative data uncovered three underlying motives that drive family historians. The search for self-understanding (who do you think you are?) was, not surprisingly, a key motive, but so was the desire to give something of value to others (generativity) and the enjoyment of learning new things and dealing with intellectual challenges. Analysis of participants' qualitative responses suggested at least four other significant although less common drivers of genealogical research, these being motives related to spiritual or meaning-of-life quests, comfort motives, making social connections and enhancing travel experiences.

In New Zealand, Theunisson (2022) interviewed 16 individuals to explore reactions to their DNA genealogical test results. She hypothesised, and found support for, the idea that DNA matches and ethnic links influenced one's sense of both social and group identity. Interestingly, this was more strongly the case among those whose DNA data contradicted their pre-test beliefs about who they were. Some experienced an 'identity crisis' while others coped by adapting their sense of self, for example by the adoption of 'multiple identities' or through re-evaluating family relationships. The literature review by Clapton (2021) discussed in the next section takes some of these ideas further for the special case of those who find out late in life that they are adopted, in many cases prompting a huge and often emotional reassessment of personal identity.

With the upsurge of interest in genealogical DNA testing and family history research, there is still tremendous opportunity for further empirical studies to assess the role that knowledge of ancestors and of previously unknown living relatives plays in mental health and wellbeing. There is much to be learned about the various ways that knowledge is shaped into personal and family narratives of success and failure, strength and weakness, resilience and vulnerability.

3. Articles Comprising Interpretive Literature Reviews

Four very different aspects of heritage are discussed and evaluated in papers by Aplin (2021); Robinson (2021); Clapton (2021) and Büster (2022). Aplin emphasises the importance of context in researching and understanding one's family history. Researching the economic, political, social and domestic behaviours, traditions and moral codes of our ancestors adds fruit and flowers to the family tree, as Aplin puts it. Such research can also engender strong feelings. It is not unusual for genealogical researchers to develop emotional attachments to places where their ancestors lived, suffered or thrived. The affective pull of heritage is also reflected in our attachments to certain family items, traditions and routines. In the wider context, we come to value objects, activities, or geographic features of the nation or nations that we identify as the source of our cultural heritage. Currently citizens from many countries are challenging which features of a nation should 'count' and be valued as heritage. This is demonstrated through, for example, rejecting once-admired monuments, or re-interpreting the importance of past 'heroes'. Whether these actions are appropriate or not, they certainly underline the sensitive role of heritage in our individual, family, local and national stories.

In her article about the parallels between religious practices and the valuing of personal heritage, Robinson discusses the ways in which ancestor research has become 'sacred practice in a secular age'. Three aspects of ancestor research are highlighted: the inheritance of 'sacred' stories and objects with familial significance; acts of pilgrimage to ancestrally significant places; and participation in 'ritual' gatherings, either with extended family or with others who share similar genealogical interests. Robinson argues that, like religion, genealogical practice can involve a spiritual element, and also like religion, can foster and strengthen feelings of identity, purpose, and belonging. As family historians, we honour our ancestors by telling their stories, continuing their traditions, making 'pilgrimages' to walk in their footsteps, and keeping alive family connections. These behaviours can contribute to our feelings of spiritual comfort and life meaning.

Büster's research and review is also about acknowledgement and honouring of ancestors, in this case from a 'deep time perspective', that is, by considering archaeological evidence from pre-literate societies and pre-historic times. Findings from the Iron Age, including domestic family items hidden in the walls of houses, are interpreted as ways of maintaining continuing bonds with the dead. Puzzling findings such as skeletal remains in which bones from several people are mixed in purposeful ways, or 'mummy bundles' in which the mummy is made up of the bones of more than one individual, raise questions as to the evolution of modern ideas of family and personhood. Büster's research review reminds us that forms of genealogy and ancestor veneration have a very, very long history. In her words, "The deep-time and global perspective presented here demonstrates that our relationships with ancestors are complex and multi-faceted, that concepts of ancestor and kin are culturally and contextually specific, and, whether positive or negative, comforting or problematic, ancestors are an ever-present and ubiquitous part of life".

Finally, Clapton's article brings us back to a modern-day issue that has loomed large since the advent of readily available DNA testing and is likely to become an even hotter topic since the more widespread use of various forms of donor conception. Clapton's paper reviews what we know about the experiences of adopted people who discover in later life that they are adopted. Without a doubt, this 'emotional bombshell' can give rise to identity conflict, a sense of betrayal and breach of trust, as individuals in this situation reflect, 'If they can keep this a secret from me, what else are they not telling me?' Some experience feelings of loss and grief as kinship knowledge, and therefore cultural and self-knowledge, are disrupted. Strong emotions like distress, anger and confusion emanate from stories told by those who discover they are not who they thought they were. While many develop ways of coping and re-shape their identities to incorporate biological and non-biological families, their stories underline the importance of giving adopted and donor-conceived children the opportunity to know about their origins from an early age.

4. Conclusions

The stories we tell about our personal, family, clan, tribal and national past all contribute to our sense of who we are—an internal narrative that shapes our self-esteem and confidence in the world. For most of us, that internal narrative is a mix of positive and negative elements—there are things we take pride in and things that shame us. To survive and prosper, psychology tells us it is better to focus on the positive, but sometimes to do that we have to first face our demons. The widespread leisure pastime of family history has, for many of us, expanded our personal narrative into the past, and given us not only an interest but a cause for excitement and joy as we discover new, colourful, even heroic characters in our family story. However, we can also feel shame or sadness as we unearth forebears who behaved badly, whose lives were 'nasty, brutish and short', or those who experienced unjust treatment, tragedy and despair. The way we balance the pride and shame, joy and sorrow, tragedy and triumph of our ancestral past will in turn shape the personal narrative of just who 'we think we are' and the family narratives that we choose to pass on to our descendants.

National histories reveal similar features. Politicians, historians, the media and other influencers present their nation's history as stories that define a 'national narrative'. As with family histories, there will be tensions between the positive and negative accounts of past events. How can these tensions be reconciled to enable constructive growth in ways that are healthy for the nation as a whole, yet acknowledge past wrongs? And, just as family historians' understanding of their ancestors' lives is enhanced by considering the broader context in which they lived, so might the understanding of world history be enhanced by the cumulative findings of family historians as they explore the lives of ordinary folk. The 'big picture' and 'little picture' approaches have the potential to be mutually beneficial to knowledge and reconciliation; a potential that has not yet been fully explored.

As well as the interrelationships between academic history research and that of family historian 'amateurs', there are many avenues (or rabbit holes!) not yet explored in researching the social and personal influences and outcomes of genealogical research. In the papers that comprise this Special Issue, many topics have been raised but not yet fully examined, for example issues relating to history education, heritage preservation, psychotherapeutic interventions, 'genealogical travel', ethical/legal issues facing family historians, and even what we mean by personal identity, family, and ancestry. As more historical documents, archaeological findings and DNA discoveries become accessible to scholars and amateur researchers alike, it is probable that interest in family history research will remain high. What we hope to have begun with this Special Issue is recognition of the opportunities to 'research the researchers', to find out more about what makes family historians tick and the potential of family history research to contribute not only to knowledge but to wellbeing.

Funding: This research received no external funding.

Acknowledgments: First: I would like to thank my co-editor Emerita Doreen Rosenthal whose support and wise counsel contributed significantly to the successful production and quality of this Special Issue. Second, thank-you to the anonymous reviewers whose time, knowledge and mental effort helped to shape and polish these published papers. Thank-you also to the Assistant Editors for their advice and assistance in ensuring that the many processes needed prior to publication were efficiently conducted in a timely manner. Special thanks are due to the Managing Editor of the Special Issue, who steered me though the processes with patience, efficiency and tact. Finally, a sincere thank-you to the authors who worked so hard to present their unique contributions to understanding the psychological impacts of family history research.

Conflicts of Interest: The author declares no conflict of interest.

References

Ainsworth, Mary D., and Silvia M. Bell. 1970. Attachment, exploration, and separation: Illustrated by the behavior of one-year-olds in a strange situation. *Child Development* 41: 49–67. [CrossRef] [PubMed]
Aplin, Graeme. 2021. Context: The role of place and heritage in genealogy. *Genealogy* 5: 58. [CrossRef]
Bhar, Sunil, and Mark Silver. 2016. Life as a Story: The Use of Digital Life Story Work in Residential Aged Care Settings in Australia. *InPsych* 38: 32–33. Available online: https://www.psychology.org.au/inpsych/2016/april/bhar (accessed on 15 February 2022).
Bifulco, Antonia. 2021. Family history and searching for hidden trauma—A personal commentary. *Genealogy* 5: 46. [CrossRef]
Bowlby, John. 1969. *Attachment and Loss*. OKS Print. New York: Basic Books.
Bowlby, John. 1982. Attachment and loss: Retrospect and prospect. *American Journal of Orthopsychiatry* 52: 664–78. [CrossRef] [PubMed]
Büster, Lindsey. 2022. From human remains to powerful objects: Ancestor research from a deep-time perspective. *Genealogy* 6. in press.
Champagne, Delight E. 1990. The genealogical search as a counseling technique. *Journal of Counseling & Development* 69: 85–87.
Clapton, Gary. 2021. Family histories, family stories and family secrets: Late discoveries of being adopted. *Genealogy* 5: 105. [CrossRef]
Freud, Sigmund. 1961. *Beyond the Pleasure Principle*. Translated by James Strachey. New York: W. W. Norton and Company.
Hershkovitz, Arnon, and Sharon Hardof-Jaffe. 2017. Genealogy as a lifelong learning endeavor. *Leisure/Loisir* 41: 535–60. [CrossRef]
Jarvis, Pam. 2021. Book Review: The Psychology of Family History. *Genealogy* 5: 39. [CrossRef]
Jarvis, Pam. 2022. Ancestral selfies and historical traumas: Who do you feel you are? *Genealogy* 6: 1. [CrossRef]
Moore, Susan M., and Doreen A. Rosenthal. 2021. What motivates family historians? A pilot scale to measure psy-chosocial drivers of research into personal ancestry. *Genealogy* 5: 83. [CrossRef]
Moore, Susan, Doreen Rosenthal, and Rebecca Robinson. 2021. *The Psychology of Family History: Exploring Our Genealogy*. Abingdon: Taylor & Francis.

Parker-Drabble, Helen. 2022. How key psychological theories can enrich our understanding of our ancestors and help improve mental health for present and future generations: A family historian's perspective. *Genealogy* 6: 4. [CrossRef]

Robinson, Rebecca. 2021. Pilgrimage and purpose: Ancestor research as sacred practice in a secular age. *Genealogy* 5: 90. [CrossRef]

Rüsen, Jorn. 1993. The development of narrative competence in historical learning: An ontogenetic hypothesis concerning moral consciousness. In *Studies in Metahistory*. Edited by Jorn Rüsen. Pretoria: Human Sciences Council.

Rüsen, Jorn. 1996. Some theoretical approaches to intercultural comparative historiography. *History and Theory* 35: 5–22. [CrossRef]

Shaw, Emma L., and Debra J. Donnelly. 2021. (Re)discovering the familial past and its impact on historical con-sciousness. *Genealogy* 5: 102. [CrossRef]

Theunisson, Catherine Agnes. 2022. The effects of DNA test results on biological and family identities. *Genealogy* 6: 17. [CrossRef]

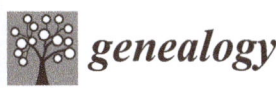 *genealogy*

Commentary

Family History and Searching for Hidden Trauma—A Personal Commentary

Antonia Bifulco

Department of Psychology, Middlesex University, London NW4 4BT, UK; a.bifulco@mdx.ac.uk

Abstract: Background: Searching family history is now popular through increased internet access coinciding with a need for understanding identity. Prior unresolved war trauma can help explain impacts on subsequent generations and the need to search for family narrative, particularly in refugee families. This paper explores the search for trauma narratives through personal family history research, with links to community groups. Method: The author's own Polish family history research provides examples of trauma and loss from World War II in Poland. This is supplemented by quotes from an existing interview study of second-generation Poles to amplify themes and indicate their wider community relevance.

Keywords: family tree; war trauma; attachment; identity; immigration; forgetting; emotional geography

Citation: Bifulco, Antonia. 2021. Family History and Searching for Hidden Trauma—A Personal Commentary. *Genealogy* 5: 46. https://doi.org/10.3390/genealogy5020046

Received: 3 March 2021
Accepted: 29 April 2021
Published: 7 May 2021

Publisher's Note: MDPI stays neutral with regard to jurisdictional claims in published maps and institutional affiliations.

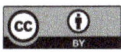

Copyright: © 2021 by the author. Licensee MDPI, Basel, Switzerland. This article is an open access article distributed under the terms and conditions of the Creative Commons Attribution (CC BY) license (https://creativecommons.org/licenses/by/4.0/).

1. Introduction

Searching for family histories seems to have increased in recent years, in part, because of the ease of accessing materials through the internet (Nicolson 2017). It mirrors an increased need for understanding familial and national identity for refugee or immigrant groups and the diaspora more generally (Brubaker 2005). This has led to the rise in companies aiding these searches (e.g., ancestry.com) and the popularity of television programmes in the UK such as the BBC's 'Who do you think you are?', exploring the family background of celebrities through documentation, historical context, and visiting places of significance. This programme often highlights collective trauma events of the last century or earlier, for example, the Holocaust (through the family stories of Robert Rinder or Helena Bonham Carter), the Partition of India (with Anita Rani), or the slave trade (with Ainsley Herriott), all these issues having social relevance today. The historical events are examined in terms of how they impacted family members at the time and their impacts for subsequent generations, including the one seeking the story. Thus, family history has evolved from simply documenting family tree members by name and date of birth/death to a more social, historical, and psychological approach, investigating family members in context and linking their stories to specific places and historical events (Nelson 2008). Often these stories include trauma-related themes.

Relatedly, an impact of 'emotional geography' (Gregory 2011) or attachment to place is invoked with the question of 'where is considered home?' given the movement of populations and diasporas (e.g., from Eastern Europe, India, or the Caribbean to the UK). This tie to places abroad can affect the social identity of the generation who first migrated, undertaking sometimes hazardous journeys and often finding adversity on arrival (e.g., racism, poverty, language, and cultural difficulties). It also can affect the second generation born in the new country in understanding family narrative, particularly those about trauma, loss, and relocation. Thus, the historical becomes personal and contemporary. It seems these individual stories strike a chord with connected communities and the larger population in gaining a greater understanding of our current ethnic populations and our recent history. This has made personal family history research into a communal and, at times, global affair. Family members can now be tracked across countries and continents (through document archives, internet, or DNA searches) and sites of family origin and possible sites of trauma events visited so that descendants can have empathy with their forebears' experience.

Genealogy embraces the interdisciplinary interests of academics who adapt traditional methods to fit this relatively new enterprise (Zerubavel 2011). From history, it borrows archival scrutiny of documentation of early family members—birth and death certificates, names on commemorative monuments, recipients of gallantry medals, etc. Historians would also be familiar with diary and informal handwritten biographical accounts and the use of photographs or family paintings to elicit information (Paperno 2004). From immigration studies emerge survey methods (e.g., census data), records of ship passenger lists, and interviews of those who settle in a new country (White 2011). Qualitative methods of data collection from psychology, such as interviews, are often combined with formal documents (e.g., case notes) for triangulation of information in pluralistic approaches (Frost and Nolas 2013). Psychologists aim to look at personal emotional impacts of past experiences, for example, immigrant journeys, including those incurred through war, separation, and loss, to seek understanding of clinical issues. Given that emotional impacts can sometimes cross generations, learning of earlier generation's trauma experiences may inform family dynamics, attachment attitudes, and impacts on children (Braga et al. 2012). Understanding both the experiences and the processes of transmission can help with understanding risk, resilience, and recovery in relation to mental health issues.

Collating family narratives can also be considered part of a therapeutic approach. In narrative therapy, for example, the aim is for the client to tell and retell their family history until a level of clarity and understanding is reached (Semmler and Williams 2000). Whilst not generally seeking external validation, the client and therapist together see how particular themes and experiences influence the client's perceptions, emotions, or behaviour. This can illuminate whether the issues to be resolved are those experienced by parents rather than the client directly, through impacts on communication, family attachment, and parental mental health (Braga et al. 2012). Even when a disorder such as posttraumatic stress disorder (PTSD) ensues, a detailed revisiting of traumatic events can release the hidden emotion if undertaken in a time and place of safety (van der Kolk 2015). By uncovering and resolving the initial traumatic experience, individuals may need to construct a narrative to communicate and work through the associated emotions. This may be aided through constructing family histories of prior events and, where relevant, linking these to historical events for confirmation. Thus, searching for family history can increase well-being and a sense of identity and belonging. This may be enhanced through recontacting lost family members or through community groups to develop communicative memory (Devlin 2020).

A pertinent question is 'why?' people seek to research their family trees and narrative, and 'for whom?' they are doing it. Many in midlife seek to pass narratives of family history onto their children to aid a sense of identity (Freedman 2015). In addition, a concern for remembrance of little-known historical events which affected the family can be a motive. When searching for commonly held political events, these family histories can also create a community narrative about traumatic events, including those of war and deportation. I consider here the impact of traumatic experiences linked to war and political events in the past and how it can affect the task of family history research and the impacts on survivors, families, and affected communities. For example, a recent study of PTSD in Poland among older-aged WWII survivors showed rates of 35%, compared to the 2% or so expected in the general population (Lis-Turlejska et al. 2018). This was despite being assessed some 70 years after the events of war trauma occurred and was more prominent where there was a lack of social acknowledgement of the experience (Rzeszutek et al. 2020). Thus, the impacts of trauma on first-generation survivors can be lifelong, with implications that recognising their stories might be a helpful intervention.

When trauma is unresolved, it can lead to many impacts including re-experiencing of the event and hypervigilance (e.g., through nightmares and flashbacks), as well as avoidance of thinking about it (even amnesia for some events), as in PTSD. This can affect other family members, such as children, when it is witnessed in the domestic arena (Zasiekina 2020). Whilst some unresolved trauma involves an inability to talk about the events, in traumatic bereavement, individuals often want to talk repeatedly about the lost person to search and yearn for reminders (Samuel 2020), although some aspects of remembering and interpreting the loss may also be impaired. Elements of blame—of self or close others—can make other relationships more toxic.

Events related to war trauma include a range of experiences involving various threats to life, involving the self, close others, and the community. In addition to *traumatic loss* (through violent bereavement or enforced separation or deportation), it encompasses *danger* associated with violence and threat of death, *entrapment* associated with enforced captivity, *deprivation* associated with starvation, and lack of shelter or enforced transportation. War trauma is thus not a single experience and often occurs over months or years. Communities and individuals may experience different levels of proximity to danger and varying 'doses' of trauma with implications for severity of clinical disorder arising across the lifespan (Felitti et al. 1998). There can also be issues of later continued traumatic stress experiences (Pat-Horenczyk and Schiff 2019; Wolmer et al. 2015) in both the first, second, and even third generations which may prolong impacts. Family history searches may be an informal way of individuals resolving their family trauma and, at times, gaining support from joining groups with similar experiences. Hopefully, this can lead to resolution and accompanying higher levels of well-being (Samuel 2020).

Understanding events of past trauma more fully may help resolve some of the impacts and issues raised in day-to-day family life. For example, the traumatised person's responses such as catastrophising over brief separations or exaggerated perceptions of neighbourhood danger and community mistrust, and fear of not having enough food may transmit to children growing up (Zasiekina 2020). Impacts may appear differently in the children or grandchildren of war survivors (Sigal et al. 1988) and include behavioural problems and problems in forming relationships (Fossion et al. 2003). This may be accompanied by an acute awareness of parental burden (Letzter-Pouw et al. 2014) as well as difficulties over a sense of identity and belonging (Cohn and Morrison 2018). Additional difficulties may be found in attachment and relationships, given the lack of a secure base (Bowlby 1988). Conversely, many individuals and families show resilience. This may be because the trauma becomes resolved in the first generation or due to resilience factors having a protective effect on subsequent family members (Bonanno 2004). Both aspects will be explored here.

2. Materials and Methods

The method employed was to collate all relevant family documents (specifically letters, diaries, and official documents) related to particular individual experiences, set these against the historical backdrop on a local level, and examine family members' responses and behaviours in relation to psychological themes. The experience of key family members described is mapped here through their letters which provide context, personal experience, and emotional response. I consider the history–psychology link in more depth as an explication of person–environment context and refugee experience.

In this paper, my focus is narrowed to my grandmother Maria, including her reaction to both her daughter-in-law Myszka's experience and her enforced separation from her only son (my father) during WWII. Emergent themes identified in relation to traumatic events include 'hidden trauma', 'remembrance/forgetting', and 'subterfuge/secrecy'. These link psychological themes to historical and political ones and speak to issues of processing trauma and traumatic loss, disclosure of events, barriers to such disclosure, and commemorating the past. I specifically consider traumatic experiences of WWII, together with internal and external barriers to disclosing trauma, which research shows can increase the risk of clinical disorders such as PTSD (see, for example, clinical approaches through van der Kolk's work as well as trauma therapy, as espoused by Judith Herman). Throughout this paper, the distinction is made between traumatic events/exposure and traumatic impacts/disorder—following DSM 5 definitions (APA 2013). Exposure to trauma is to actual or threatened death, serious injury, or sexual violation. Exposure includes direct experience, witnessing the event in person or learning of the event to a close person, or exposure to aversive details of the traumatic event. This includes the experience of war. Impacts of trauma, in contrast, include emotional response, symptoms such as PTSD, and unresolved trauma related to fragmented recall or inability to disclose the experience.

Another more general theme identified is 'emotional geography' which is about attachment to a place where we call home and a sense of belonging. This speaks to our sense of identity and is relevant to those deported or refugee and the feelings of dislocation which can impact future generations. This relates to the second element of the method which extends the single-family case study to include quoted experience from other WWII Polish families in UK second-generation interviews (White and Goodwin 2019). This set of 28 interviews was originally arranged by themes, and those relevant to this analysis include 'parents, grandparents, and trauma' and 'long lost family in Poland, Belarus, and Ukraine'. Many of the interviewees had parents who were forcibly deported by Russian troops from Poland in February 1940 to Siberian labour camps in ethnic cleansing (Davies 2015). They lived in inhumane conditions until release, after Russia joined the allies when they were sent on long journeys for refuge in British Commonwealth countries across three continents. These stories are not widely known (Devlin 2020). Their inclusion here is to provide some direct interview quotes which resonate with the themes identified to indicate potentially unresolved trauma from events not publicly acknowledged. They also serve to broaden the range of the single case study to a community group.

3. Results

3.1. My Family Story Outline

My grandmother Maria, my father's first wife Myszka, and my father Jurek were living in Warsaw at the outbreak of WWII, my father having married Myszka a year earlier. Warsaw was badly bombed under invasion and suffered harsh Nazi occupation for the next five years. Whilst this affected all the local population, it was the harshest for the many Jews of the city (and those transported in from other areas and countries, of around half a million people), who were restricted to a small, overcrowded ghetto area (equivalent to 10 city blocks). They suffered multiple deprivations and, ultimately, death either through being sent to concentration camps or through the harsh suppression of the Warsaw Ghetto uprising in 1943 (Ringelblum 2015). This was the first of two civilian uprisings; the second in 1944 was also harshly suppressed. My grandmother in Warsaw lived through the occupation in her own home, unaware of Myszka's secret activities for the Polish Resistance. Myszka was caught and sent to Auschwitz where she died a year later. I have some of her story from her wartime letters to my father and my grandmother's letters to my father after the war and more from her nephew in Poland who made sudden contact recently. My father's close cousin Staś was also conscripted into Polish forces at the start of the war but disappeared in the first months of occupation. Several years later, after the war, his death in the massacre of 20,000 Polish officers in 1940 at Katyn was known by the families involved. However, responsibility for the massacre was delayed for nearly 50 years.

My father, newly conscripted into the Polish army in 1939, was ordered to make his way to France to join the allied forces. He came to England in 1943, was recruited by Special Operations Executive (SOE), Churchill's 'secret army' (Crowdy 2016), and trained as a paratrooper to be dropped behind enemy lines in Warsaw to aid the Uprising in August 1944. At the last minute, this plan was countermanded by Churchill, and Warsaw faced the destruction of German troops and then occupation by Soviet Russia (Davies 2004).

This information is taken from my mother's notes of discussion with my father, as well as from photographs and official documents. A sad corollary was that on VE day celebrations 1945, Poles were forbidden from being represented in UK commemoration, under Russian pressure. They were viewed by Russians as deserting their country in order to fight with British forces (fulfilled with great heroism and as the largest foreign fighting force against fascism). My parents met on VE day in an English midland town, my English mother smitten by the sad but handsome Pole who felt unable to join in the celebrations.

3.2. My Grandmother's Traumatic Experience

My grandmother Maria's experience of traumatic events during the war in Poland is first revealed in her letters to my father in England some months after the war in 1946. This was the first she knew of his survival, having last heard from him in France in 1942, and she made an official search in January 1946 to alleviate her 'torment of uncertainty', as evidenced by the following letter:

> Dear Sir,
>
> I would earnestly like to ask you if could let me know whether you have any news about the fate of my son, Jerzy Tadeusz Czechowski, born 16 October 1913. The last communication I had from him was on 10 August 1942. In Spring 1943, thanks to your information, I knew that he was alive and well, since then there has been no news. Please forgive me if I am causing you any inconvenience, even more so that you yourself are suffering, but the torments of uncertainty, which I am undergoing because of the lack of information about my only son, may explain my boldness. I will be everlastingly grateful for any, even the most trivial, information. I thank you in anticipation. (Bifulco 2017, p. 170) (Page numbers of the letters below are also from this reference).

Maria managed to make contact with her son Jurek in February 1946, and they make contact after nearly four years of silence and her 'terror and despair'.

> My dearest son, my dearest Jurek
>
> I'm beginning my letter with your words: today I lived through the most beautiful day of my life. For nearly four years I have not had a single word from you. I will not dwell on the years of German occupation because there aren't enough words of terror and despair, but all that was as nothing compared to the two months of August and September in 1944. On 1st October after capitulation, those who were left alive had to wander away looking for somewhere to live. I spent half a year in a village 25km from Krakow. On 23rd March 1945 I returned to Warsaw which was in ruins. By some miracle our house survived although it was very badly damaged, without a roof, but it could be used. Of course, I left with only the clothes I was wearing and returned to completely nothing. (p. 171)

She writes later that year (April 1946) about her living conditions.

> I live in just one room, the one facing the street. The rest of the dwelling has been taken over by the family of a minor railway official. It consists of five people who even before my return, took over the whole part of the house that had not been devastated. I had to repair the room facing the street, that had been ruined during the Uprising, before I could move in on 8th July 1945. For three months I had to take advantage of the hospitality of neighbours. You probably know that your flat was plundered in 1939 and the furniture was sold. Not even the smallest keepsake was left. Whereas my flat was robbed of everything after the Warsaw Uprising. So we are both very poor. (p. 172)

My grandmother is also the one who had to update my father by letter of family losses.

> Myszka, your wife, was sent to Auschwitz in October 1943 and from that time there has been no news of her. From our closer family, Leszek, Mirek's brother, died in action in 1939 and Uncle Janek's two sons Włodek and Jurek were shot in the forest. Also, no signs of life from Staś, the son of Aunt Julia and Walek. The rest of the family are alive and managing somehow. (p. 171)

Maria has the courage to tell Jurek of Myszka's fate in a later letter in May 1946.

> Jurek my dear, I didn't want to add to your troubles, so I didn't tell you the whole truth straight away. Myszka is no longer alive. I received her death certificate from Auschwitz. She died on 10 January 1944. She stopped coming to see me about one and a half years before this and cut off any contact with our whole family. (p. 173)

The bearing of such bad news is in itself vicarious trauma, both for the giver and receiver of the information. I do not know how my father received this news or how painful it was for my grandmother to write it. However, it is not easy to disclose by means of a slow postal system nor yet to receive news of loss similarly by letter.

My grandmother writes about her own health also in May 1946.

> As for my hearing, there is probably no hope of a cure. Firstly because of the cold in unheated apartments (seven winters already) I had chronic catarrh in my ears and finally I lost my hearing during the Uprising when I was hit by a so called 'szafa'. The worst thing under the sun. It is a missile of compressed air. This was the only thing I was afraid of during the war and of getting into the hands of the Germans.

> My hair is now completely grey and I wear horn-rimmed spectacles. You probably wouldn't recognise me, in addition I've become a cry baby, like a child. (p. 173)

This latter comment is the only one in her letters about her own state of mind and her distress and anxiety. She is generally optimistic, buoyed up by a strong religious faith and good support from her sister-in-law and niece. She writes to Jurek as follows:

> I would so like to write and write about many things at length. I ask but one thing of you, my dear son: be of good cheer, believe in Providence, throw yourself completely on God's mercy and it will lead you to a happy ending. For the whole year, every day, a Mass is celebrated for your good intentions and not a day passes without my praying for you. I hope that by the end of this year we can be together. (p. 171)

Thus, despite describing her traumatic events, she also shows she is able to retain optimism, gratitude, and faith. This, together with support from close family members who similarly survived in Warsaw, seems to have sustained her. My father also seems to have been resilient after the war, having the benefits of a loving marriage and family and a safe place to settle in the UK despite some practical hardships. My grandmother joined the family in the UK in 1958, four years before she died, having already contracted cancer and at a time when restrictions on travel were eased. My father was unable to return to Poland due to the Cold War restrictions, and his next visit was in 1965 for a family holiday, 25 years after leaving and a first family reunion. My sisters and I were brought up in the English Midlands amidst an active Polish community.

I do not recall my grandmother ever speaking of her war experiences in the household when she came to England in 1958. Neither do I have evidence that she was *unable* to speak of them. She did not display any mental health issues although physically she remained deaf, and the cancer that killed her was already spreading by the time she came to live with us.

Her traumatic events comprised violent losses of those close to her and enforced separations with no knowledge of survival, the experience of bombing leading to deafness, physical hardship regarding food and heating, as well as the hostile occupation of her city, heightened during the Warsaw Uprising which started in her street. In addition, she became a refugee for some months, being forced to evacuate the city and taking no belongings. This would also have been true for the rest of the city population. In terms of the impact of trauma, her letters show she is able to outline some of her experience in writing, showing practical coping and retaining close contact with family nearby. She also holds onto her religious faith. Even though she says she has become fearful, there is no obvious indication of either PTSD or depression. This indicates likely resilience.

The traumatic events my grandmother experienced seem not to have transmitted generationally even though she lived her final years with her son and grandchildren. Of course, this was more than 10 years after the end of the war, and it is possible that this time period allowed for some trauma resolution. I am aware of no mental health difficulties for her when she came to England, nor in the second generation of the family. When trauma is argued to transmit across generations, this is usually evidenced by substantial relating problems (Shamtoub 2013) and negative world assumptions (Bachem et al. 2019). These do not seem to have been present in my family among the second generation who have had long-term marriages, raised children successfully, and had productive careers. It also needs to be acknowledged that traumatic experience does not necessarily transmit, for example, some studies of Holocaust survivors showing no effects relative to peers (Van Ijzendoorn et al. 2003) and others showing a positive role for resilience factors such as positive family communication (Giladi and Bell 2013). Resilience to trauma has been identified as the more usual response, although this is less for 'corrosive environments' which are long lasting (Bonanno 2004) and also for war trauma (Kessler et al. 2017). The sort of resilience which is relevant is loving family, stable temperaments, social support, and strong community and religious ties (Fonagy et al. 1994). It was also notable that my grandmother had a happy and settled childhood, this occurring at a time of relative political peace pre-WWI. Yet, she had experienced prior trauma as an adult, through WWI in which her young husband fought with the allied Russian troops, and the Germans occupied Warsaw prior to armistice. She lived through the Russian Revolution of 1917 when, with her army officer husband and infant son, she had to urgently escape to Romania, and through the Polish–Bolshevik war in 1920 during which fighting reached the gates of Warsaw and in which her husband died, aged 33. Thus, she and her young son would have been exposed to six years of war, but she seems to have survived this with little evidence of long-term impacts of trauma. The concept of 'steeling' may apply whereby individuals learn survival skills through prior testing (Rutter 1985). This is therefore a positive message about surviving trauma.

However, this was not always the case with other people whose parents had experiences of war trauma. The issue of war trauma and its impacts was explored in the Invisible Poles study in the second-generation interviews (White and Goodwin 2019) (page numbers of quotes below refer to this document). This provides examples of those who experienced impacts of trauma in their parents. Adelaide describes her own family history, discoveries which helped explain her father's PTSD as follows:

> My father died thirty-four years ago, and six years ago I started my research. And the first thing I did was get his documents from the Ministry of Defense. Then, of course, I found out where he came from—I looked it up on the map, and I asked the Red Cross to look for his family, because he said they were all gone. And I did a lot of reading about that, you know, the history around there, and learned a great deal about those people's experience. And I understand very much why he was ... He had post-traumatic stress disorder. You know, like many older Polish people who've been through those experiences do. And after three years the Red Cross found his family. Well, what was left of his family. (White and Goodwin 2019, pp. 26–27)

A few of those interviewed also identified impacts of trauma in their parents, which were undiagnosed and untreated due, in part, to the barriers on disclosure as showing 'weakness'. Natalie says the following:

> Post-traumatic stress is post-traumatic stress. Whatever the stress was, and the trauma. It's somehow not even acknowledged. My mum suffered from a mental breakdown ... It's more than just a stiff upper lip, because, deep inside, they are crying out themselves. But we must not let that be shown, because it would be a weakness. (White and Goodwin 2019, p. 33)

These quotes support the research evidence of trauma having long-term effects on clinical disorders and show the barriers to seeking help. Resolving traumatic experiences relates to both recalling and the ability to disclose events. Barriers to this can be both psychological and environmental. These are further discussed.

3.3. Remembering Trauma

Remembering traumatic experiences can be problematic for survivors. Responses such as PTSD involve a combination of over-remembering (such as in flashbacks and nightmares) and amnesia for the events (avoidance of thinking about the trauma and blocking of thoughts and feelings) (APA 2013). There are complex reasons for individuals being unable to recall or disclose trauma, these being both psychological and physiological (van der Kolk 2015). Reports of silence in survivors of WWII regarding their traumatic experience are common, as described by their children (Letzter-Pouw et al. 2014). Brief factual reports may be provided but not detailed accounts of what happened with associated feelings. It is argued that such disclosure can only occur when the individual feels truly safe—yet those with unresolved trauma never feel this safety even when their new circumstances are benign (van der Kolk 2015).

Accounts of parents being unable to discuss their war trauma are given by the next generation in relation to the WWII experience. Natalia (White and Goodwin 2019) states the following:

> You don't know the secrets that a lot of these people kept. There's been research done on the children of Holocaust survivors. Surely there must be some on the children of people who survived the Stalinist regime? My grandparents died en route- coming out of Siberia—and their daughter, my aunty, had to bury them where they fell. That's not a very pleasant thing to do for a person who is a teenager ... that must be awful at whatever age you are. And thinking where are you going to end up, or are you going to end up anywhere? Where's your next meal going to be? (White and Goodwin 2019, p. 32)

This was echoed by Adelaide as follows:

> My father never talked about his background, like many of them don't. He was very secretive. He told us his family in Poland were all gone. I went in 2016 for the first time and found he had a wife in Poland and a son, my half-brother. They were no longer alive sadly. But my nephew is there ... they are so happy that I found them. It's been wonderful to connect I feel a strong connection ... I feel a blood connection with them in Ukraine. (White and Goodwin 2019, p. 43)

Iza reports that others do not necessarily want to hear about the trauma.

> I suppose that's left me with [a view that] the less war the better. Appreciating that people don't just survive, they have things that go on. All the relatives that didn't survive but also the impact on the next generation. Some of the reading I've done, I've liked it where you read what the people my generation have been saying ... And I thought it was very interesting, watching the story being told in Poland. Because people don't necessarily want to hear it again. I want to hear it. But some of my generation think 'Not again. It's too much.' Not in a horrible way, but it's very heavy, and they've heard it, whereas I haven't. So, you can see, some of them are just like, 'Now we're here,' they're saying, 'Now we're in the EU and why are we still talking about that?' (White and Goodwin 2019, p. 35)

There are of course many events that occur in a war which are later hidden and which would be uncomfortable to hear. Psychologists can consider how being unable to disclose traumatic events affects the individual and their families. Researching family history can open doors on such events for individuals and increase understanding of family members' behaviour.

3.4. Forgetting, Secrecy, and Subterfuge

Family members are often in ignorance of events of war trauma through external barriers to disclosure. As already described, my grandmother lived through the Warsaw Uprising and five years under the German occupation of Poland with its reign of terror. There was in fact widespread and secret resistance in Poland at the time, which curtailed individuals speaking to each other about clandestine activities, as well as lack of information about family members killed or separated and fighting abroad. The Home Army in Poland had the largest European resistance to the Nazis under occupation, with a large portion of the population involved (Bor-Komorowski 2010). This was highly organised and highly secret, with individuals risking their lives to take part, including children and adolescents. Families would not necessarily know if members were involved. Secrecy ensured the safety of others but precluded any family discussion of events which can also curtail the resolution of fear and trauma (Karski [1944] 2012). Often family members disappeared suddenly—either killed or imprisoned or sent to concentration camps for their activities.

My grandmother would not have known about her daughter-in-law Myszka's activities even though they were in close contact. Myszka worked in a Red Cross hospital but was secretly a liaison worker for the Polish resistance. Historical analysis now shows the life expectancy of a liaison worker, most of whom were women, was 3 months during the occupation of Poland (Davies 2004). Myszka's role was uncovered during a random roundup of civilians by German soldiers. She was arrested, imprisoned, and sent to Auschwitz where she died a year later. Family members did not know of this until after the war, as already described. I only recently heard the details of Myszka's wartime activity when her nephew in Poland, who I had never met, emailed my sister unexpectedly with the following account:

> She was involved in the Resistance. In her work with the Red Cross she managed to get into contact with Jurek. In 1942, at a łapanki [random round-up] she was stopped with false documents and carrying false papers. She was transferred to the Gestapo and sent to the Pawiak prison. Because our family was wealthy (before the war we owned a sugar factory) we tried to pay for her freedom. There was no chance, because she was considered public enemy of the Reich No. 1, and a political prisoner. The only thing was to commute the death penalty to being sent to the concentration camp in Auschwitz. She was sent to the camp at the end of August 1942. (Bifulco 2017, p. 115)

Thus, throughout the war, the fate of many close family members was unknown which curtailed personal or official mourning. This too can contribute to unresolved trauma and long-lasting psychological effects on survivors (Samuel 2020).

Events might also be hidden for family reasons. I only learned as a young adult about Myszka and the fact that my father had been married before the war in Poland. He subsequently met and married my mother after the war in England. His first marriage was kept secret from us as children on the pretext that it would be too confusing for us but likely due to my mother's jealous nature. I was able to find out a lot about Myszka from her letters sent to my father during the war, which had been carefully preserved and now newly translated. My grandmother had also preserved the German death certificate issued at Auschwitz. My research indicated that Myszka was a vibrant, funny, energetic young woman who wrote lively letters to my father in France during wartime, making light of the awful conditions in Warsaw under the Nazis. We have copies of the photographs she had sent to him in France. However, no mention was made by her of her activities as a secret liaison worker in the Polish home army. It seemed sad to me that the family did not honour her memory and talk about her in the family. Similar to other deaths in concentration camps, there is no grave or personal memorial to her.

Silence about wartime trauma can be due to enforced secrecy, as required sometimes in war, but also due to selected secrecy agreed in families for more emotional reasons. In my family, it does not seem to have had a deleterious effect on family life, but I suspect it was hard for my father not to acknowledge her, and as children, I think we would have liked to have known.

3.5. Public Forgetting

There is another side to the forgetting of traumatic events, which is also external to the individual, involving the ability of society more generally to speak of community traumatic events. This can be politically motivated and can relate to a lack of social acknowledgement of trauma which can result in worse psychological outcomes on a community scale (Lis-Turlejska et al. 2018). At certain times, the state can suppress open discussion of events either for reasons of ideology or expediency or due to state secrets legislation. This occurred in the Cold War with suppression of historical WWII information during Stalinist times and later. Certain events were deemed never to have happened. I will describe one here which affected my family—the massacre at Katyn, Russia.

This massacre of over 20,000 Polish officers, now officially recognised as a war atrocity committed by the Soviets in 1940, was only finally acknowledged by President Gorbachev with the fall of communism. It then became public knowledge that the order for the killings was signed in 1940 by Stalin. The massacre occurred in April 1940 when Russia had secretly signed their non-aggression pact with Hitler, an alliance downplayed in their subsequent fight against German fascism (Maresch 2010). Responsibility for the Katyn massacre was officially denied in the Soviet Union, despite an official UN investigation involving international scientists, which took place when the mass burial site was first uncovered by the advancing German army in 1943. There was substantial evidence of the likely Soviet perpetrators, fully documented in UN and Red Cross reports. There were also eyewitnesses—both locals and Poles who escaped (Karski [1944] 2012).

The coverup of Katyn even extended to the Western world. Fear of Stalin in the 1950s meant that Poles in the UK (around 200,000, who, as combatants, could not return to Poland without reprisals) were not allowed to speak openly about the massacre and its perpetrators, nor to erect a commemorative monument in central London. The UK government did, however, allow a monument to be raised in a small cemetery in West London, local to where many Poles lived at that time. However, they were instructed by both the British and Soviet governments to add no details to the wording of the monument inferring culpability to avoid a diplomatic incident. The Poles therefore simply engraved the black monolith as 'Katyn 1940'. Even this caused some official outrage since, given the time and place, it implicated Russian involvement. Katyn could not be openly discussed in Poland under Soviet control. This lack of social acknowledgement and barriers to mourning and remembrance must have affected families of officers killed in the massacre, both in the short term through not knowing of the deaths and longer term through lack of public acknowledgement and discussion. My father's cousin Staś suffered that fate; we now know he was shot in the back of the head in the Katyn forest on his 25th birthday. My father always believed it to be a Russian atrocity—given he had met eyewitnesses in England. I was therefore brought up knowing about Katyn, but Staś's mother Julia and the family did not learn of his death until some seven years later, as evidenced by my grandmother's account of family members lost in April 1946. Not knowing the outcome of loss is a factor in chronic and unresolved mourning—imagining the person might be alive or in pain or distress is a constant barrier to being able to accept a loss as final (Samuel 2020).

The cause of the Katyn massacre was not officially recognised until 1989, many years after Julia's death. She did not live to see the new Polish republic raise monuments and a recent museum to the dead at Katyn, as well as create an internet archive with photographs of each man lost with his name and date of birth. This would have been true for the families of all those killed. These names are also now listed in metal or stone in churches and cemeteries in Warsaw. This provides a highly individualised approach to remembrance. I have visited these and seen the name of Staś (Stanislaw Leinweber) accurately listed. His picture, familiar from our mantelpiece during my childhood growing up, is the same now shown on the internet. It is noted that such personalised information could not have been collated in previous decades before the internet or while the iron curtain was still in place. Sometimes, a time delay gives a greater chance of collecting and displaying information to provide further knowledge of family events.

Issues surrounding remembering and processing war trauma are complex and will vary by individual and family but with some processes hindered by lack of social and political acknowledgement. Yet, these can change over time with restrictions and secrecy lifted so that over generations people can finally have trauma acknowledged. This makes an ongoing search for family history capable of finding new facts over subsequent decades.

3.6. Emotional Geography and Belonging

Distances can be measured differently in relation to emotional geography where far-away places may be experienced as close because of emotional and family ties (Rubinstein and Parmelee 1992). Attachment involves the 'holding in mind' of the attachment figure and this may also extend to places of emotional importance. Therefore, a place considered to be home may be held as a close event even though difficult or even impossible to visit. These barriers are amplified when the place lost is also linked to a lost time when conditions were different. This can lead to a sense of yearning for a lost home.

In terms of the Polish WWII experience, many of the Poles who were deported from their homes in eastern Poland by Soviet troops found these were later annexed into Lithuania, Belarus, or Ukraine. My own family's original home in eastern Poland is now in Belarus. For family history, this can complicate the finding of family documents and may create further barriers of language and borders as countries can become more or less distant depending on politics and transport opportunities. When I was a child, Poland was considered far away from the UK. This was due to travel times (36 h by train) and because, at times, during the Cold War, visiting there was impossible. Later in the 1960s, when visits were possible, there was a substantial red tape with visas and other documentation required, together with the obstacle of armed soldiers monitoring the borders from West to East Germany, with long queues, all cars being searched, and great nervousness in case of stowaways or contraband being seized. It was at that time virtually impossible to make phone calls to Poland, all correspondence being by letters, and these being prone to censorship and with slow progress to delivery. Therefore, Poland was effectively distant. Now it takes two hours airplane travel from Heathrow, close to my home in West London, to Warsaw. Until recently, we were in the same European Union with freedom of travel for work or leisure. Warsaw can easily be visited for a weekend holiday and other parts of Poland are now popular holiday destinations for the British and other Europeans.

Attachment to place ideally conveys a sense of a safe haven (Hernández et al. 2007). For many, it will be the place where they live or were born, and individuals can have more than one such home without feelings of dissonance. However, for others when their home is a foreign country where their parents or grandparents were born and where they cannot easily return it can set up a sense of yearning. This may be for a geographic location, but also of a time prior to trauma experienced and recognised as unreachable. Thus, for immigrants and refugees, 'home' may be a country far away, which, for second and subsequent generations, may be one never visited.

The second-generation WWII family survivors interviewed talked about home and family in Poland and their parents' attachment to (or indeed fear of) their original homes. Aniela speaks of her parents first going home as follows:

(First visit to Poland 1974): *Mum and Dad desperately wanted to see all of it . . . . And they took them to the places they were born, in the Ukraine . . . so they went to see the places where they would have grown up in. Mum was desperately wanting to see that. I think she had to do that. Its a form of closure almost, she's been to see her birthplace. They have no documents, no birth certificates or anything.* (White and Goodwin 2019, p. 29)

This is echoed by Adelaide.

Poland was a place of danger . . . my father created it as a place of danger . . . And I was afraid of it. I didn't get to Poland until 2006. I went to Warsaw and Krakow . . . what a wonderful place. I was amazed at how young the population was because I only knew old Polish people. (White and Goodwin 2019, p. 49)

The question of belonging in a country can depend on the level of integration of immigrant communities, as well as with second and third generations accepting the new country as home.

Although the first WWII generation is now being lost due to age, documenting the long-term impacts of trauma on families and succeeding generations is important for understanding the ongoing mental health and well-being of populations in relation to historical events. Survivors of war trauma commonly have difficulties communicating their experience (van der Kolk 2015); therefore, later family members may only have a basic idea of what occurred yet still suffer from impacts. Sharing narratives in some form among this group may be of important benefit for resilience and well-being (Fivush and Zaman 2011). Refugee populations who have additional negative experiences on arrival may also exhibit suspiciousness of services in their new country and therefore have barriers to help-seeking.

Natalia makes the connection between current refugees and her parents' experience and speaks of atonement.

> When you see Syria and the atrocities now, you think that could be my parents, that could be my family. And the idea that some of the places there's fighting now, they are actually the places where they were given succour. They were looked after. The Kazhak women were seen as wonderful. My Dad went through Persia, Iran . . . .but the war is still there and people still living in horrific circumstances. I suppose that's the humanitarian aspect of me wanting to know more. And, of course, somehow atone for what my parents went through. (White and Goodwin 2019, p. 32)

4. Conclusions

The information provided here about personal family history has been selected to illuminate issues related to experiences of war trauma in families. The focus has been on whether such experience can be openly discussed, with barriers including psychological ones related to posttraumatic response, political ones including denial of atrocities, and secrecy including subterfuge during war or events hidden under state secrets legislation. These all relate to experiences undisclosed at the time, or even for some duration of time, but which can be later discovered in family research connected to historical analysis. It is generally recognised that the impact of traumatic events is lessened when people are able to talk about the trauma, receive social acknowledgement, and complete family narratives of loss and danger (Herman 1992; Lis-Turlejska et al. 2018).

A key message is that exposure to war trauma does not always lead to disorder and is not necessarily transmitted across generations and that emotional survival and resilience are common. The key distinction to be made is of traumatic events (which can be personal or public) and impacts of trauma which are personal and psychological, although potentially experienced by communities. Many more individuals experience traumatic events in their lifetime than experience disorders such as PTSD, implying some degree of resilience is to be expected. However, there may be other impacts of trauma for war survivors, including those surrounding attachment insecurity negative worldviews and other common disorders such as depression or anxiety. However, even where these are present, we do not necessarily know how to attribute such impacts; for example, an individual who lives through war may also have experienced early life abuse in his/her family creating vulnerability. This alone or the combination with adult war trauma may have a 'dose' effect on the disorder (Felitti et al. 1998). Alternatively, someone surviving war trauma may later suffer other personal trauma through bereavement or violent attack in peacetime, making attribution of causal connection to disorder complex.

Not all family research will necessarily be as positive as mine in showing resilience or indeed in finding a wealth of relevant information. My contact with Polish Jewish Holocaust survivors in the UK suggests the desire for searching their history is hampered by the extermination of all family members, their lack of knowledge or connection to their pre-war homes, and their lingering distrust of countries where genocide occurred. For them, meaningful narratives may also lie in the communicative memory of their generation of survivors and publicly archived materials (Devlin 2020).

The effort of tracing a family narrative and learning of the lives of our parents, grandparents, and beyond can give a sense of completeness, enhanced identity, and produce unexpected links to present life. For example, tracing talents or professional interests across generations (many writers in my family) or finding relatives who look alike through shared

DNA (the son of my second cousin who looks like my father), or visiting streets and seeing houses, where family lived over a hundred years ago, can bring deep sense of connection to people and places. It is a lengthy and absorbing task to undertake family history research but can lead to finding treasure as well as trauma.

Funding: This research received no external funding.

Institutional Review Board Statement: Ethical review were waived for this study all family documents owned by the author.

Informed Consent Statement: Individuals referred to all deceased. Consent from family members received.

Conflicts of Interest: The author declares no conflict of interest.

References

APA. 2013. *Diagnostic and Statistical Manual of Mental Disorders (DSM-5®)*. Arlington: American Psychiatric Association.
Bachem, Rahel, Johanna Scherf, Yafit Levin, Michela Schröder-Abé, and Zahava Solomon. 2019. The role of parental negative world assumptions in the intergenerational transmission of war trauma. *Social Psychiatry and Psychiatric Epidemiology* 55: 745–55. [CrossRef]
Bifulco, Antonia. 2017. *Identity, Attachment and Resilience: Exploring Three Generations of a Polish Family*. London: Routledge.
Bonanno, Goerge. 2004. Loss, Trauma and Human Resilience: Have we underestimated the human capacity to thrive after extremely aversive events? *American Psychologist* 59: 20–28. [CrossRef] [PubMed]
Bor-Komorowski, Tadeusz. 2010. *The Secret Army. The Memoires of General Bor-Komorowski*. Barnsley: Frontline Books.
Bowlby, John. 1988. *A Secure Base: Clinical Application of Attachment Theory*. London: Routledge.
Braga, Luciana, Marcelo Mello, and Jose Fiks. 2012. Transgenerational transmission of trauma and resilience: A qualitative study with Brazilian offspring of Holocaust survivors. *BMC Psychiatry* 12: 134. [CrossRef]
Brubaker, Rogers. 2005. The 'diaspora' diaspora. *Ethnic and Racial Studies* 28: 1–19. [CrossRef]
Cohn, Ilana, and Natalie Morrison. 2018. Echoes of transgenerational trauma in the lived experiences of Jewish Australian grandchildren of Holocaust survivors. *Australian Journal of Psychology* 70: 199–207. [CrossRef]
Crowdy, Terry. 2016. *SOE: Churchill's Secret Agents*. Oxford: Shire Publications Ltd.
Davies, Norman. 2004. *Rising '44' The Battle for Warsaw'*. Basingstoke and Oxford: Pan Books, Macmillan.
Davies, Norman. 2015. *Trail of Hope: The Anders Army, an Odessey across Three Continents*. Oxford: Osprey Publishing.
Devlin, Julia. 2020. In Search of the Missing Narrative: Children of Polish Deportees in Great Britain. *The International Journal of Information, Diversity, & Inclusion* 4: 22–35. [CrossRef]
Felitti, Vincent, Robert Anda, Dale Nordenberg, David Williamson, Alison Spitz, Valerie Edwards, Mary Koss, and James Marks. 1998. Relationship of Childhood Abuse and Household Dysfunction to Many of the Leading Causes of Death in Adults: The Adverse Childhood Experiences (ACE) Study. *American Journal of Preventive Medicine* 14: 245. [CrossRef]
Fivush, Robyn, and Widaad Zaman. 2011. Intergenerational narratives: How collective family stories relate to adolescents' emotional well-being. *Aurora. Revista de Arte, Mídia e Política* 10: 51–63.
Fonagy, Peter, Miriam Steele, Howard Steele, Anna Higgitt, and Mary Target. 1994. The Emanuel Miller Memorial Lecture 1992: The theory and practice of resilience. *Journal of Child Psychology and Psychiatry and Allied Disciplines* 35: 231–57. [CrossRef] [PubMed]
Fossion, Pierre, Mari-Carmen Rejas, Laurent Servais, Isy Pelc, and Siegi Hirsch. 2003. Family approach with grandchildren of Holocaust survivors. *American Journal of Psychotherapy* 57: 519–27. [CrossRef]
Freedman, Jean. 2015. *Whistling in the Dark: Memory and Culture in Wartime*. London: University Press of Kentucky.
Frost, Nollaig, and Sevasti-Melissa Nolas. 2013. The Contribution of Pluralistic Qualitative Approaches to Mixed Methods Evaluations. In *New Directions for Evaluation*. Edited by D. M. Mertens and S. Hesse-Biber. Manhattan: Wiley, pp. 75–84.
Giladi, Lotem, and Terece Bell. 2013. Protective factors for intergenerational transmission of trauma among second and third generation Holocaust survivors. *Psychological Trauma: Theory, Research, Practice, and Policy* 5: 384. [CrossRef]
Gregory, Derek. 2011. *The Dictionary of Human Geography*. Chichester: John Wiley & Sons.
Herman, Judith. 1992. *Trauma and Recovery*. London: Pandora (HarperCollinsPublishers).
Hernández, Bernardo, Carmen Hidalgo, Esther Salazar-Laplace, and Stephany Hess. 2007. Place attachment and place identity in natives and non-natives. *Journal of Environmental Psychology* 27: 310–19. [CrossRef]
Karski, Jan. 2012. *The Story of a Secret State. My Report to the World*. London: Penguin Classics. First published 1944.
Kessler, Ronald, Sergio Aguilar-Gaxiola, Jordy Alonso, Corina Benjet, Evelyn Bromet, Graca Cardoso, Louisa Degenhardt, Giovanni de Girolamo, Rumyana V Dinolova, Finola Ferry, and et al. 2017. Trauma and PTSD in the WHO World Mental Health Surveys. *European Journal of Psychotraumatology* 8: 1353383. [CrossRef]
Letzter-Pouw, Sonia, Amit Shrira, Menachem Ben-Ezra, and Yuval Palgi. 2014. Trauma transmission through perceived parental burden among Holocaust survivors' offspring and grandchildren. *Psychological Trauma: Theory, Research, Practice, and Policy* 6: 420. [CrossRef]

Lis-Turlejska, Maya, Szymon Szumiał, and Iwona Drapała. 2018. Posttraumatic stress symptoms among Polish World War II survivors: The role of social acknowledgement. *European Journal of Psychotraumatology* 9: 1423831. [CrossRef]

Maresch, Eugenia. 2010. *Katyn 1940—The Documentary Evidence of the West's Betrayal*. Stroud: The History Press.

Nelson, Alondra. 2008. The factness of diaspora. In *Revisiting Race in a Genomic Age*. New Brunswick: Rutgers University Press.

Nicolson, Paula. 2017. *Genealogy, Psychology and Identity: Tales from a Family Tree*. London: Routledge.

Paperno, Irina. 2004. What Can Be Done with Diaries? *The Russian Review* 63: 561–73. [CrossRef]

Pat-Horenczyk, Ruth, and Miriam Schiff. 2019. Continuous traumatic stress and the life cycle: Exposure to repeated political violence in Israel. *Current Psychiatry Reports* 21: 71. [CrossRef] [PubMed]

Ringelblum, Emmanuel. 2015. *Notes from the Warsaw Ghetto: The Journal of Emmanuel Ringelblum*. Auckland: Pickle Partners Publishing.

Rubinstein, Robert, and Patricia Parmelee. 1992. Attachment to Place and the Representation of the Life Course by the Elderly. In *Place Attachment. Human Behavior and Environment (Advances in Theory and Research)*. Edited by Irwin Altman and Setha Low. Boston: Springer, vol. 12.

Rutter, Michael. 1985. Resilience in the face of adversity: Protective factors and resistance to psychiatric disorder. *British Journal of Psychiatry* 147: 598–611. [CrossRef]

Rzeszutek, Marcin, Maja Lis-Turlejska, Aleksandra Krajewska, Amelia Zawadzka, Michał Lewandowski, and Szymon Szumiał. 2020. Long-Term Psychological Consequences of World War II Trauma Among Polish Survivors: A Mixed-Methods Study on the Role of Social Acknowledgment. *Frontiers in Psychology* 11: 210. [CrossRef] [PubMed]

Samuel, Julia. 2020. *This too Shall Pass: Stories of Change, Grief and Hopeful Beginnings*. Penuguin: Random House.

Semmler, Pamela, and Carmen Williams. 2000. Narrative Therapy: A Storied Context for Multicultural Counseling. *Journal of Multicultural Counseling and Development* 28: 51–62. [CrossRef]

Shamtoub, Yasi. 2013. *Intergenerational Transmission of Trauma and Attachment in Adult Children of Iranian Immigrants*. San Diego: Alliant International University.

Sigal, John, Vincenzo Dinicola, and Michael Buonvino. 1988. Grandchildren of survivors: Can negative effects of prolonged exposure to excessive stress be observed two generations later? *The Canadian Journal of Psychiatry* 33: 207–12. [CrossRef]

van der Kolk, Bessel. 2015. *The Body Keeps the Score: Mind, Brain and Body in the Transformation of Trauma*. London: Penguin.

Van Ijzendoorn, Marinus, Marian Bakermans-Kranenburg, and Abraham Sagi-Schwartz. 2003. Are children of Holocaust survivors less well-adapted? A meta-analytic investigation of secondary traumatization. *Journal of Traumatic Stress* 16: 459–69. [CrossRef]

White, Anne. 2011. *Polish Families and Migration Since EU Accession*. Bristol: The Policy Press.

White, Anne, and Kinga Goodwin. 2019. *Invisibe Poles: A Book of Interview Extracts*. London: University College London. Available online: https://discovery.ucl.ac.uk/id/eprint/10070108/ (accessed on 4 March 2021).

Wolmer, Leo, Daniel Hamiel, Tali Versano-Eisman, Michel Slone, Nitzan Margalit, and Nathaniel Laor. 2015. Preschool Israeli children exposed to rocket attacks: Assessment, risk, and resilience. *Journal of Traumatic Stress* 28: 441–47. [CrossRef] [PubMed]

Zasiekina, Larysa. 2020. Trauma, Rememory and Language in Holodomor Survivors' Narratives. *Psycholinguistics* 27: 80–94. [CrossRef]

Zerubavel, Eviator. 2011. *Ancestors & Relatives: Genealogy, Identity, & Community*. Oxford: Oxford University Press.

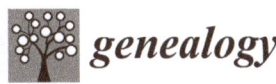 genealogy MDPI

Concept Paper

Context: The Role of Place and Heritage in Genealogy

Graeme Aplin

Independent Researcher, Wahroonga, NSW 2076, Australia; graemeaplin@optusnet.com.au

Abstract: Genealogical research often focuses to varying degrees on the family tree and the ancestors that inhabit it, often ignoring, or at least downplaying, broader issues. There is, however, much scope for broadening the research by adding leaves and flowers to the fruit (the people) on the tree. The broader context to a person's ancestry is often intriguing and enlightening, providing background information that places the people in their environments, perhaps explaining their actions and lifestyles in the process. Two aspects of this context are dealt with here. The first aspect relates to the place in which each person lives, in other words, to their geographical environment, both natural and social or human made. Secondly, their personal heritage is considered: this includes the most important items in their lives, perhaps inconsequential to others but with long-term meaning for them and quite possibly for their descendants. Other broader aspects of heritage may well be relevant, too.

Keywords: family history; context; environments; homelands; heritage

Citation: Aplin, Graeme. 2021. Context: The Role of Place and Heritage in Genealogy. *Genealogy* 5: 58. https://doi.org/10.3390/genealogy5020058

Received: 13 April 2021
Accepted: 13 June 2021
Published: 16 June 2021

Publisher's Note: MDPI stays neutral with regard to jurisdictional claims in published maps and institutional affiliations.

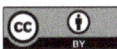

Copyright: © 2021 by the author. Licensee MDPI, Basel, Switzerland. This article is an open access article distributed under the terms and conditions of the Creative Commons Attribution (CC BY) license (https://creativecommons.org/licenses/by/4.0/).

1. Introduction

Aplin (2002, p. 1) begins the Introduction to his book on heritage with the following passage:

We are all products of our personal and collective pasts, including those of our forebears and of local, ethnic, religious, and other groups to which we belong.

That, of course, also applies to our ancestors, those people on our family trees: their pasts are also, by extension, our pasts. Hence, finding out about all of those pasts is important in understanding our own past and present. However, as Jacobs states:

'Kids don't get inspired simply by learning the names, dates, and birthplaces of their ancestors. The key is the family narrative'. (Jacobs 2017, p. 50)

Two interrelated aspects of those pasts and of that narrative are the environments in which each person lived periods of their life, often termed their homeland(s), and what they saw as being the most important aspects of their heritage. Each of these two aspects will be treated separately, but remember, they are in a very real sense intertwined. However, important as they are, they will not help us understand the character of any individual fully, as the most personal aspects are not normally documented in the majority of the sources with which this paper deals, except perhaps in newspapers and the like, in military records, and, perhaps less fortunately, in court and hospital records. So, more traditional genealogical research is still crucially important, and the approaches suggested here are no replacement for it but an elaboration on it. Perhaps it is true to say, without being too negative, that:

Amateur local and family historians face a steep learning curve to analyse their data, view it in the framework of broader world and national history, and report their findings in ways that do justice to context. (Moore et al. 2021, p. 8)

While I am writing from an Australian cultural and family background, with my ancestors coming from the British Isles, the comments and suggestions that I make can be applied much more widely. Details of what is possible and what approaches need to be taken will, of course, differ from place to place.

2. Context for the Family Tree

Family history researchers will often need to rely on living people's memories, so get in while those memories are intact and use what written evidence there is, such as letters or diaries, often kept very privately by still-living relatives. While 'studying family history usually begins with us talking to our nearest relatives, listening to their stories, piecing together the relationships, achievements, tragedies, triumphs and scandals' (Moore et al. 2021, p. 5), this need not be the end of the family history project. Those more personal aspects will become even more meaningful if seen in their environmental and heritage contexts.

Many genealogists and family-history researchers undoubtedly already do some, or indeed much, of what is suggested in the following sections. If so, they are down the road from a family tree to a family history or, if concentrating on an individual, to a historical biography. The latter two outcomes can be much richer than a basic family tree and more rewarding for the reader, as well as for the researcher and the study's living subjects.

The steps suggested in this paper will lead to a much more complete and informative outcome than would creating a bare family tree. If the people are the fruit on the tree, the contextual and circumstantial material alluded to in what follows can add the flowers and foliage. The matters in question can be broadly seen as environmental and heritage related. Environmental issues can be economic, social and political, as well as being related to the physical environment, the last including the built environment, whether rural or urban. All are part of a person's 'homeland', as is their heritage.

Family history is here seen to be set within the context of one or, probably, very many local, regional and even national histories. The extended genealogical or family history research outlined and advocated here will thus place the family members within a much broader context. It will hopefully be informative and even entertaining, while helping to explain relationships and outcomes along the branches of the family tree. The tree will, as a result, provide much more than merely a list of people and the bare relationships and lines of descent between them. It must be added, though, that what you learn about individuals may not always be positive or welcome news. Why, for example, was someone on my family tree banished from England to Rhodesia last century? Unfortunately, I do not know the answer. If I did know the answer, or that to any other possibly sensitive question, I would need to be extra careful in using it in my family history.

Of course, the geographical context and related heritage matters will be different for each person on the family tree, at least to a minor extent. The differences may become major as more distant branches of the tree are considered. As a result, the extra research needed to make these extensions could be very great and time consuming, but the outcomes may well be very rewarding and warrant that time and effort. In fact, with international migration and now (at least pre-COVID-19) such easy movement between places and cultural environments, any individual may have existed within a number of very different contexts at different stages in their life, and as compared to their close relatives. How far you extend your research is up to you, but you probably will not go as far as implied in the title of Jacobs' very readable book: *It's All Relative: Adventures Up and Down the World's Family Tree* (Jacobs 2017). As he states, we—all human beings, in fact—are all related if you extend the 'family tree' far enough, but what value of 'n' will you use to limit your tree to 'nth' cousins?

Some of the possible sources will be familiar to many people doing their family trees, but some will not be familiar to everyone. First and foremost, talk to surviving relatives, and even friends and acquaintances of the main characters focused on in this endeavour. Do this while you still have the opportunity, especially as related to older people, such as parents and grandparents. Ask them about places and relevant heritage features, as well as about the people as such. They will often be a fount of information that will help give context to the people on the family tree. What was their life like? Where did they live? Where did they meet? Did they move around, perhaps even migrating to a different country? If so, what was their new environment like for them?

As made clear by Kyle (2011, p. 20): 'asking questions, critical questions, leads to the best kind of family story writing'. She also makes the point that photographs, maps and other illustrative material may also be invaluable (Kyle 2011, p. 20). These materials, along with words, may be available in the various sources dealt with in this paper. You may or may not feel comfortable, however, with Kyle's use of the terms 'easy' and 'very easy' in the titles of her very helpful books (Kyle 2007, 2011). Darby and Clough (2013) outline a model of the family history research process, in which stages increase in depth and difficulty. They also state that the steps may be repeated for each ancestral line.

Karskens notes a word of caution, pointing out that information on females on the family tree will frequently be harder to obtain than information on males, especially in the past (Karskens 2020, p. 17). If the place of residence or other association is known, this should not matter, as the same sources can be used as you would for a male. However, it may be more difficult to determine what place that was, especially for pre-marriage portions of a female's life. At the same time, as Karskens goes on to state in subsequent pages, historical writings and official records can tell you a lot about general attitudes to marriage and other relationships, such as the frequent marriage of older men to very young girls/women in early New South Wales (p. 332ff). As Jacobs puts it:

> Even if we find the names of women from our past on various government documents, we often know little beyond that. Women are frequently ciphers, lacking stories, feelings, opinions. (Jacobs 2017, p. 232)

Similar comments can be made about ethnic and other minority groups. For example, it is very difficult to find information on many Australian Aboriginal people, especially those of the 'stolen generations' taken from their biological parents and placed in institutions or fostered by Europeans. The genealogist's task is made even more difficult by Aborigines not having surnames in the European sense until they became part of European Australian society. After a conversation with a former nurse at an Aboriginal mission, followed by a lot of help from Mr Google, I found a number of North Queensland Aboriginal people named 'Aplin', my surname. They had taken Aplin as their surname when they lived and worked on a large property owned by a great-uncle of mine. By contrast, there are very good records of the convicts transported to Australia in the late 18th and early 19th centuries: for a long time, Australians were loath to admit they had convict ancestors, even loath to try and find out if they did, but in recent decades having such ancestors has become almost a thing of great pride.

As will become very evident, if you are lucky, there is likely to be an enormous amount of material available to you, so this may be an appropriate place to quote Kyle (2011, pp. 21–22) once again:

> [Writing] a family history is a unique process. However, it has at its heart a challenge familiar to most writers: how to rein in and shape a coherent story out of the overabundance of collected data now residing on our desks, in our computers and even under our beds!

All of the sources mentioned in the following sections may contain vital, or at least interesting, information. Just as importantly, however, they may well point you in the direction of other sources. Indeed, the total collection of sources may seem to you to be like a spider's web or a tangled mass of kelp fronds. Do not despair; untangling things can be fun, even if frequently frustrating, certainly time consuming. However, as Moore et al. (2021) state:

> Standards of proof are important, and the dedicated genealogical researcher looks to 'triangulate' data, especially where there are ambiguities or inconsistencies in information collected. (p. 5)

Unfortunately, inconsistencies and ambiguities are all too common, particularly as much of the information is likely to be subjective, rather than objective. When you interpret the information and draw conclusions, another source of subjectivity enters the scene: this is inevitable, but care needs to be taken to be as objective as possible.

One of the respondents in the research exercise of Moore et al. sums up the nature of family history as follows:

> It is like working on a giant jigsaw puzzle and filling in small sections at a time. There are a few holes I dream of filling one day before I die. Each new piece gives me satisfaction. I am constantly amazed by the information which is available online . . . Gradually, you can build up a picture of someone's life. (Quoted in Moore et al. 2021, p. 73)

3. Sense of Place: The Environmental and Geographic Context

Every person on any family tree will have lived, worked, played and travelled in particular places and environments, their 'homelands', to use current genealogical jargon. They will also have met each other, if that is relevant, in a particular place. They may have moved many times, or they may have stayed in the same place for all of their life, perhaps in the same place as their ancestors. Finding out even a little, and that may be all that is possible, about that place or those places will add to the understanding of the people involved. In some cases, knowing of a major move, even to a vastly different country through either voluntary or forced migration, will help understand the people and the lives they lived. There may, of course, have been dramatic changes between the period before the move and that after it.

Increasingly, genealogy studies will rely in part on DNA analyses. The results of these will often point to otherwise unknown and unanticipated branches on the family tree. At least in a broad national or regional sense, the results may open up connections with places not previously envisaged as relevant. They may also reveal unpleasant aspects of the person's ancestry, and privacy becomes of paramount importance here. Of course, individual ancestors and relatives are probably unlikely to be revealed, but at least environmental contexts and heritages are highlighted for investigation.

How does one find out about a particular place? In particular, how does one find out about a place at some time in the past? Lynch's book is titled *What Time is This Place?*: its main theme is summarised in the opening sentence of the dust-jacket blurb: 'In the personal image of a city the sense of place is meshed with the sense of time' (Lynch 1972). In an earlier work (Lynch 1960), he deals with how we conjure up images of places, specifically cities. The sense of place and the sense of time both involve the set of features that make a place recognisably different, easily identifiable and memorable (Aplin 1987). Together, they are the place's character at a particular time, summing up the nature and ethos of the place and leading to an accepted group or individual image of that place at that time. So, you will want to know what a place was like when the person on your family tree was there, when it was their 'homeland', and that certainly may not be what that place is like today.

If the places being investigated are in a nation or involve an ethnic group speaking a language other than your own, or other than one in which you are reasonably competent and comfortable, you will need assistance with translation. This applies to all of the potential sources mentioned in the following paragraphs. It will very likely also make communications with libraries and other officials more difficult. However, there is hope, as one respondent in the study of Moore et al. shows:

> Because half of my family history has been in Europe—mostly in the Russian Empire of the 19th century, I have learnt to read handwritten birth, death and marriage certificates in Russian. I had studied some Russian before that, but not at a high level. This has been an enjoyable and rewarding challenge. (Quoted in Moore et al. 2021, p. 33)

I imagine this genealogist would also tackle the other sources referred to in this paper if they were in Russian, handwritten or printed.

If you are lucky, a local history of the relevant place will have been written. This may, or may not, be useful, however. Some local histories focus narrowly on the people who lived there, and your family-tree characters may or may not be featured. However, that local history may well not give much, if any, indication of what that place was like at various times. An example that I have seen is Weeks (2004), a local history of Lydford in the United Kingdom; it is strong on personalities but not so strong on the sense of place at various times. Alternatively, Karskens (2020) is a wonderfully detailed history of both the people and their environment on the Nepean–Hawkesbury River, west of Sydney in the late 18th century and the 19th century. Sometimes, there will be a well-researched work dealing with all the major places in a region, such as the wonderful volume on California (Abeloe 1966) or the 'Places' section in the Australian Bicentennial History volume *Events and Places* (Aplin et al. 1987). Of course, specific local histories or these broader collections may not cover all of the time periods relevant for your family tree or family history research. They need not, though, specifically mention the characters on your tree, as it is the environment and geographic context for each of them that is the key issue being addressed. Papers in journals such as this one will frequently be relevant, for example, Davies (2021) who uses the diary of an important ancestor as a key source. Online indexes are a key point of entry to such material. Academic theses are yet another potential resource, although possibly harder to find and use.

In some cases, town or city directories may be of assistance, even going as far back as the Domesday Book covering England and parts of Wales in 1086, now available online. As another more recent Australian example, many directories of Sydney published in the 19th century list occupants street by street, including both residences and businesses (for example, Low 1845). This might give an idea of not only the address of your person of interest, but also of the general nature of their surroundings and of the broad type of people who were their neighbours. Censuses may also give an indication of the broader population characteristics of a particular town or rural area.

At least a general overview of a country or region can be gained from reading geographic and historic works and even travel guides, such as the *DK Eyewitness Travel* series or the *Lonely Planet* series. Depending on the places of interest to you, you may gain much more from such works, especially if those places are better known and more important. As with any of the sources mentioned in this paper, the most rewarding aspect of these general works is that they may well point you in the direction of further research and to more specific resources.

Being the 21st century, one cannot ignore Wikipedia and search engines such as Google. Relevant local history, genealogical and community groups often have pages on Facebook and the like, too. Wikipedia has entries on surprisingly small and unimportant places, as well as on larger towns, cities, regions and countries. Most Wikipedia entries are frequently being checked, corrected and added to, though this may be less likely for smaller centres. There will also be entries on people and local institutions. By and large, this source is reliable, though checking against other sources is always a good idea, if possible. The same is true for the other sources already mentioned and those that follow, particularly as they have often relied on personal memories, and these are not always reliable.

Google and other search engines can lead you to the official sites of local government bodies, and these frequently include a reasonably sized section on local geography and history. Other bodies, both volunteer-based ones, such as historical societies, and more official ones, such as business groups, farming organisations, military units and educational institutions, are all likely to have websites that can be checked for relevant content. So, too, can religious, sporting, arts and leisure-oriented organisations.

Local and broader scale newspapers and magazines may also be useful, especially if they have been included in library collections, which makes them more accessible, and, hopefully, they will have been indexed. In Australia, we are lucky to have Trove, the website of the National Library of Australia, which makes it possible to easily search all the newspapers in their collection, many surprisingly small and local ones, as well as books and academic papers and theses. If you do use Trove or an equivalent, or look into the collection in any other library or archives, you might need to actually go there and use the material on the spot. Some items listed on Trove, for example, are available online, but far from all of them are, and physical borrowing of material is unlikely to be possible if a distant library is involved. Two other advantages of a library visit are that you might gain ideas for other sources by browsing the shelves and that the staff will almost invariably be of great assistance.

Finally, if at all possible, visit the places of interest that have connections to people on your family tree. Basu (2005) writes of the ways that a new form of travel referred to as 'genealogical tourism' can contribute to developing a sense of place, the place in which your ancestors once lived. When it comes to a distant past, visiting the place of origin might provide insight into such matters as the difficulties of farming or the remoteness of village life. A visit will be particularly rewarding if a large number of your tree-family relate to the one place, less so if they have been widely scattered over many places. You should be able to get a feel for the environment and heritage (next section) of a place. Most valuably, you may be able to speak with people with a knowledge of your ancestors and relatives. Struckland (2018), for example, writes of his urge to visit Norway to follow up on some of his Norwegian ancestors. In his case, these ancestors came to the USA as migrants. Many people in that country, and in others such as Australia and Canada, for example, have migrant forebears and can profit greatly by following up on the homelands of these people, possibly visiting their places of origin, as Struckman did. Two papers by or involving Solène Prince also deal well with genealogical or ancestral tourism: Prince (2021) and Mehtiyeva and Prince (2020). The *Journal of Heritage Tourism* is also a possible source more broadly and is particularly relevant to the following section.

It is important to remember that it will not be present conditions that are of interest, but conditions at times relevant to the lives of people on your family tree. Many Australians came to their new country from war-torn Europe or conflicts in Southeast Asia, the Middle East or Africa, at least in the days of Australian governments being more sympathetic to refugees. Friends of mine with Hungarian or Czech family backgrounds, for example, have commented to me on how great the changes have been since they left, or from what their parents and grandparents have spoken about.

Archaeological work might also be very relevant, though not necessarily that involving ancient sites. Archaeologists have, in recent decades, realised increasingly that their work can assist our understanding of historic times, perhaps quite recent ones. A friend of mine was reminded of a recent archaeological dig in Tasmania, where they uncovered artefacts from the convict road station set up when convicts were building the Heritage Highway. This was of interest to her because her convict ancestor was in a road gang building this highway and at one point was given 35 lashes for sitting down on the job. She is going to visit this dig spot next time she goes to Tasmania. Purely by coincidence, a 19th-century ancestor of my wife was also a convict in the same general area, very likely at the same time, and we found out on a visit to the most relevant town in Tasmania that his sentence was truncated, and he became a police officer supervising later convicts. I need to liaise with my friend and look for connections. This is the kind of outcome from site visits and local records that can add significantly to a family history.

4. Heritage

'Heritage' can have many meanings. One interpretation of a person's heritage relates to their cultural background and is both wide reaching and akin to their homeland or certain of the kinds of environmental contexts referred to in the previous section. Another interpretation, and the one used for the following section, relates to particular sites (and sights) and individual objects that are important to the person with whom you are concerned. These personal heritage items may be included in the broader heritage, or they may not. For example, family historians may view as part of their personal heritage the towns, farming areas and even houses where their ancestors lived, the churches where they married and the high streets where they shopped. One described to me the sense of excitement she felt in locating the Powis castle estate in Wales where her fourth great-grandfather had run the flour mill, the town of Westbury in Wiltshire where her second great-grandfather stole 12 rounds of cheese (and was transported to Van Diemen's Land)

and the St Michael and All Angels' Church in Haworth where several of her ancestors were baptised by the Reverend Patrick Bronte, father of the Bronte sisters.

In recent decades, heritage in a societal context has become much more important in public debate, and governments at all levels in many nations have legislated to protect at least some key elements of it. Heritage occurs on all scales from the global World Heritage List, through national, state (or equivalent) and local government levels to the very local and even personal levels. However, heritage in the broader sense goes far beyond what is inscribed on official lists. A person's heritage reflects their homelands at various periods in their life, hence the strong link with the previous section, but also their cultural background and also their individuality and personality. As with homelands, it is the heritage of the relevant time for each person that needs to be researched, and this may be very difficult to do in terms of a lack of evidence of earlier views of heritage, or those of different countries.

The official registers concentrate on heritage sites that are considered important under agreed criteria concerning natural environments, cultural or built environments or a mixture of the two. Items are placed on the lists because they are deemed to be of importance under those criteria, and at the relevant scale, for present and future populations. There is often a historical element in the reasons for inscription, but not necessarily so. Obviously, not everyone in the relevant cohort will agree on the decision to list; after all, we all have different views on our environments and the objects within them. Once listed, heritage items are given legal protection from changes that detract from their listing criteria, although there are frequently loopholes that do allow change and development, even elimination.

Particular items of natural heritage relevant here might be a coastal area where your person of interest surfed, a national park where they bushwalked or studied the wildlife, a river where they fished or a view they adored. In the cultural heritage field, various sites and individual buildings might be important: where your subject went to school, worshipped, holidayed or met their partner might be especially meaningful to them. There are an almost infinite number of reasons why a place or object might be of great importance to any individual.

There are also some official lists referring to intangible and moveable heritage items and these are the objects likely to be cared for in museums and libraries. Also included in some cases are folk dances and music, other social events, belief systems, endangered languages and on and on it goes. Perhaps the most notable intangible heritage lists are the UNESCO Memory of the World Register (UNESCO 2012) and the list for the Convention for the Safeguarding of the Intangible Cultural Heritage. Sometimes items on these and similar lists will have a clear relationship with a place, frequently with a nation or region. The included items may well have importance for people on your family tree. We have already mentioned libraries, but local museums, especially history museums, may also give assistance in finding what is/was of personal importance to people on your family tree. More generally, historical museums will very likely give important pointers to what the local area was like at various times in the past, thus linking us back to the previous section of this paper.

In fact, the definition of what constitutes 'heritage' is an individual, subjective matter depending on a person's background, life experience and personality, although groups of people, perhaps defined on a socio-economic, cultural or ethnic basis, may share many aspects of their perceptions. In similar fashion, the definition of 'heritage' in any particular country depends on local historical, social and cultural circumstances. Within any nation, the 'official' or 'accepted' definition is frequently that of some dominant group. In other words, the concept of 'heritage' is appropriated by that group as one more manifestation of its dominance in politics and national debate. Some 'ownership' of at least part of the officially recognised heritage of a country is important to many groups to help manufacture and maintain their group identity, for example, indigenous peoples, migrant groups, religious denominations and local communities. One example is the difficulty the Basque population in Spain is having in getting its heritage recognised at the national level or, even more pointedly, the troubles the Rohingya people have in Myanmar. Fernández (2020) touches on the need for migrants to the US from Galicia (another minority population in Spain) and their descendants to establish and maintain ties with their ancestral homeland and to understand their heritage. She deals with the value of visits to that homeland, something raised earlier in this paper. Closer to my home, the heritage of the Australian Aboriginal and Torres Strait Islander peoples is finally being increasingly recognised as being a crucial element in our national heritage. It is absolutely crucial to people in those groups and would be an essential part of any family history involving them.

An individual featuring on a family tree or in a family history will have their own bundle of heritage items important to them, even if not always to anyone else. Often, some very personal item or experience will feature front and centre in a person's understanding of their heritage. This could be a childhood toy, such as a bunny, a child's blanket or an early item of clothing, things that seem trivial to anyone else. It might be a pet cat or dog, a favourite holiday location, a school or sporting centre or, later in life, a favourite car. Such items could be unique to the individual and help define who they were and what their personality was like. As such, they may add important information on the life of the person(s) concerned and thus increase the value of your family tree.

One can then look at increasingly broad areas and the heritage items involved in those expanding spheres. It is important to be aware of the fact that an individual's understanding of the importance of heritage items may well be quite different from the official bodies' views. A person may have seen something that escaped the official list as being of crucial importance for them, while they may also think that a listed item is unimportant. In the present context, an individual's view of heritage is important, not that of some government body. Again, sources beyond the official ones might well be central to understanding what heritage items mattered to the person on your family tree, and, preferably, why they mattered. It is also crucial to remember that heritage from a cultural background very different from that of a person's present location may be most important. As an example, British settlers in Australia brought a vast amount of British heritage with them, including placenames, food and customs. They even imported plants, animals and birds to remind them of 'home'. Some of these plants and animals subsequently became detested pests in their new home. More recent immigrant communities in Australia have also retained many features of the culture and heritage of their countries of origin, greatly enriching Australian life as a result.

As stated above, any significant concern with heritage, at least officially, is quite recent, basically increasing from the early 19th century in voluntary bodies, such as the National Trusts in various nations, then being taken up by governments at all levels. The success of these listing processes is very variable. The point here, however, is that there were not usually equivalent heritage lists in earlier times, so other sources will probably need to be used. The same items as are now on the lists, as well as others that have been demolished or irrevocably altered since the time of interest to you, could be the very ones that mattered most to the person you are wanting to study. As well as that, people's views on what are and are not important items have changed over time. Some of the sources treated earlier under the 'Environment' section are also key for heritage.

One type of heritage listing that may be particularly relevant in the family history and genealogy context is the World Heritage Committee's category of 'Cultural Landscape', first used officially by that body in 1987 (Aplin 2007, pp. 427–28). Such listings, beginning in 1992, involve a marriage between physical landscapes and human occupation and alteration of them. Compared to most World Heritage sites, Cultural Landscapes are broader, both spatially and conceptually. According to the World Heritage Committee (WHC):

> There exist(s) a great variety of landscapes that are representative of the different regions of the world. Combined works of nature and humankind, they express a long and intimate relationship between peoples and their natural environment. ... To reveal and sustain the great diversity of interactions between humans and their environment, to protect living traditional cultures and preserve traces of

those which have disappeared, these sites ... have been inscribed on the World Heritage List. (WHC 2004; Aplin 2007, p. 430)

In many ways, a Cultural Landscape can be seen as analogous to the genealogist's 'homeland'. All examples inscribed on the World Heritage List have full descriptions and justifications available at the WHC website, whc.unesco.org (accessed on 15 June 2021). The WHC website currently (April 2021) lists 115 inscribed Cultural Landscapes, as well as giving much information on the concept, and on the criteria and processes involved in listing (WHC 2021). Some sites are basically agricultural regions, while many others are much harder to categorise, being 'various mixtures of architecture, sacred or religious sites, traditional land use, and spiritually important landscapes' (Aplin 2007, pp. 436–37). Yet, others relate to routes of cultural importance.

If your homeland of interest happens to be located in one of these inscribed sites, you are very fortunate and can use the information provided. If it does not, then these examples provide a template for what you might do, presumably on a smaller scale, to write up a description of your homeland of interest.

5. Conclusions

As Karskens notes: 'Any historical approach that ignores human emotions will fail to see the forces that compelled people's movements, interactions, strategies and behaviours' (Karskens 2020, p. 326). She goes on to stress that lives in the past were often less than smooth going. The approaches I suggest in this paper are, in a sense, taking things the other way around. The 'forces' Karskens refers to are to a large degree encapsulated in a person's environment and their heritage. Knowledge of these aspects will help understand both the 'movements, interactions, strategies and behaviours' and perhaps extend an understanding of the subject's personality and emotions. However, these more abstract aspects of a person's life in the past are bound to need some more personal source of information to be fully understood in relation to that personality and those emotions.

The aim of the approaches and use of sources dealt with above is to add spice to your family tree, to make it much more than simply a visual representation of family relationships across the decades and centuries. Instead of the bare branches with a few names on them, you can have something more like a highly decorated Christmas tree. Assuming you have a family tree that goes back a considerable period of time and extends to more distant relationships, perhaps including people living in different 'homelands', there will be a great deal of work involved in turning the family tree into a family history. It will be very rewarding, though, and an excellent hobby to keep the mind sharp, as well as something of great value to share with other family members and to leave for future generations, who will, hopefully, add to it as time goes by. As Australian feminist Anne Summers says of her family history endeavour:

> I loved the moment of triumph whenever a sliver of information fell into place, when I cracked the challenge of a library catalogue or when I made the connection between two seemingly unrelated events. (Summers 2009, p. 42) Moreover, you may even be able to add some entertainment value: when the author sourced his father's Australian Army records, he found the entry 'Son born' (me), and the pencilled query someone had added 'Married?'. My father had omitted to tell the Army that he married my mother on his previous home leave, almost exactly nine months previously.

Funding: This research received no external funding.

Institutional Review Board Statement: Not applicable.

Informed Consent Statement: Not applicable.

Conflicts of Interest: The author declares no conflict of interest.

References

Abeloe, W. N. 1966. *Historic Spots in California*, rev. 3rd ed. Edited by M. B. Hoover, H. E. Rensch and E. G. Rensch. Stanford: Stanford University Press.

Aplin, G. 2002. *Heritage: Identification, Conservation, and Management*. Melbourne: Oxford University Press.

Aplin, G. 2007. World Heritage Cutural Landscapes. *International Journal of Heritge Studies* 13: 427–46. [CrossRef]

Aplin, G. J. 1987. Sense of time, sense of place. Paper presented at Conference of the Sydney History Group, Sydney, Australia.

Aplin, G., S. G. Foster, and M. McKernan, eds. 1987. *Australians: Events and Places*. Sydney: Fairfax, Syme & Weldon Associates.

Basu, P. 2005. Macpherson Country: Genealogical identities, spatial histories and the Scottish diasporic clanscape. *Cultural Geographies* 12: 123–50. [CrossRef]

Darby, P., and P. Clough. 2013. Investigating the information-seeking behaviour of genealogists and family historians. *Journal of Information Science* 39: 73–84. [CrossRef]

Davies, B. 2021. Re-turning to the event of colonisation in New South Wales. *Genealogy* 5: 2. [CrossRef]

Fernández, N. 2020. Constructing National Identity Through Galician Homeland Tourism. *Genealogy* 4: 1. [CrossRef]

Jacobs, A. J. 2017. *It's All Relative: Adventures Up and Down the World's Family Tree*. London: Oneworld Publications.

Karskens, G. 2020. *People of the River: Lost Worlds of Early Australia*. Sydney: Allen & Unwin.

Kyle, N. 2007. *Writing Family History Made Very Easy: A Beginner's Guide*. Sydney: Allen & Unwin.

Kyle, N. 2011. *How to Write and Publish Your Family History in 10 Easy Steps*. Sydney: New South Publishing.

Low, F. 1845. *The City of Sydney Directory for 1844–5*. Sydney: Facsimile reprint by the Library of Australian History.

Lynch, K. 1960. *The Image of the City*. Cambridge: MIT Press.

Lynch, K. 1972. *What Time Is This Place?* Cambridge: MIT Press.

Mehtiyeva, A., and S. Prince. 2020. Journeys of research, emotions and belonging: An exploratory analysis of the motivations and experience of ancestral tourists. *Scandinavian Journal of Hospitality and Tourism* 20: 85–103. [CrossRef]

Moore, S., D. Rosenthal, and R. Robinson. 2021. *The Psychology of Family History: Exploring Our Genealogy*. Abingdon: Routledge.

Prince, S. 2021. Affect and performance in ancestral tourism: Stories of everyday life, personal heritage, and the family. *Journal of Heritage Tourism*. Available online: https://www.tandfonline.com/doi/full/10.1080/1743873X.2021.1883033 (accessed on 12 February 2021). [CrossRef]

Struckland, R. 2018. A U.S. traveler's urge to see Norway is all in his genes: As genealogy rises in popularity, more tourists are being inspired to explore their ancestral homelands. *The Washington Post*, September 20.

Summers, A. 2009. *The Lost Mother*; Melbourne: Melbourne University Press. Available online: www.trove.nla.gov.au (accessed on 15 June 2021).

UNESCO. 2012. *Memory of the World*. Paris: UNESCO Publishing; Glasgow: Harper Collins.

Weeks, B. 2004. *The Book of Lydford, an Saxon Borough*. Tiverton: Halsgrove.

WHC (World Heritage Committee). 2004. Cultural Landscapes. Available online: whc.unesco.org (accessed on 11 June 2021).

WHC (World Heritage Committee). 2021. 'Cultural Landscapes', Available from the WHC Website under 'Activities' and then 'Cultural Landscapes'. Available online: whc.unesco.org (accessed on 11 June 2021).

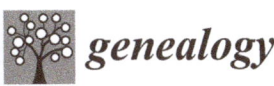

Article

What Motivates Family Historians? A Pilot Scale to Measure Psychosocial Drivers of Research into Personal Ancestry

Susan M. Moore [1,*] and Doreen A. Rosenthal [2]

1. Department of Psychology, Swinburne University of Technology, Melbourne 3122, Australia
2. School of Population and Global Health, The University of Melbourne, Melbourne 3010, Australia; d.rosenthal@unimelb.edu.au
* Correspondence: smoore@swin.edu.au

Abstract: Participation in family history research may be a passing phase for some, but for others, it is a recreational pursuit exciting passionate intensity that goes beyond idle curiosity or short-term interest. In this paper, we explore some of the underlying motives that drive amateur genealogists, including the search for self-understanding, the desire to give something of value to others and the enjoyment of the many intellectual challenges that this hobby can provide. Using data accessed from an online survey of 775 Australian family historians, we developed a reliable and valid measure of the intensity of these psychosocial motives and used research participants' qualitative data to suggest four further motives of interest for future research and measure development.

Keywords: genealogical motivation; family history and identity; family history and altruism; family history and curiosity

Citation: Moore, Susan M., and Doreen A. Rosenthal. 2021. What Motivates Family Historians? A Pilot Scale to Measure Psychosocial Drivers of Research into Personal Ancestry. *Genealogy* 5: 83. https://doi.org/10.3390/genealogy5030083

Received: 21 July 2021
Accepted: 13 September 2021
Published: 15 September 2021

Publisher's Note: MDPI stays neutral with regard to jurisdictional claims in published maps and institutional affiliations.

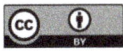

Copyright: © 2021 by the authors. Licensee MDPI, Basel, Switzerland. This article is an open access article distributed under the terms and conditions of the Creative Commons Attribution (CC BY) license (https://creativecommons.org/licenses/by/4.0/).

1. Introduction

Family history has always been a popular pastime, whether it involves drawing up family trees or recording stories from the past. In recent years, the availability of so many records online, and the possibility of finding DNA matches, has escalated this 'hobby' into a worldwide craze. Amateur genealogists can spend many hours and often a significant amount of money drawing up family pedigrees and researching the lives of their forebears. What is the attraction? Sometimes the reasons are practical and short-term, such as validating a family story, writing a eulogy or helping a child with a homework assignment. However, a surprising number of amateur genealogists find themselves 'addicted', such as one who described her hobby as *"an all-consuming passion that's hard to walk away from ... "* (Moore et al. 2021, p. 2). What psychosocial factors might motivate this intense interest, raising it to something beyond an occasional recreational pursuit? The major aim of this study was to develop a measure of the nature and intensity of psychosocial motives that drive family historians to persist in their quest to discover more about the ancestral past.

One motivator for exploring family history, popularised by the 'Who do you think you are?' television programs, is the search for self-understanding—finding your 'true self' or identity through knowing more about where you come from, not only in terms of individual ancestors but in relation to cultural heritage (e.g., Bottero 2012; Darongkamas and Lorenc 2008; Walters 2020). The notion of identity, popularised by psychologist Eric Erikson (1980) refers to our sense of who we are and where we're going; a personal narrative that we create as we experience the vagaries of life and come to understand our strengths, weaknesses and the forces that have shaped us. McAdams (2001) argues that this personal narrative provides a sense of unity, meaning and purpose in life. Bottero (2015) extends the idea further to include not only self-understanding, but cultural identification and connectedness to others. Additionally, understanding the lives of our ancestors awakens us to the history of how people lived in the past, a lens through which understanding of one's present circumstances may be enhanced (Kramer 2011a; Lambert 1996; Parham 2008).

Some family historians do their 'identity work' by very specifically searching for a lost relative, biological parent or sibling (Hertz 1998; Müller and Perry 2001; Sobol and Cardiff 1983), or for clues about their medical history and inherited risk factors (Birt et al. 2014; Spector 2013). Others take a more exploratory approach, collecting stories of ancestors and thinking about them in relation to a general family narrative or personal identity development. For example, discovery that one's ancestral 'story' involves overcoming hardships by direct action can provide personal inspiration in current difficult times, while noting the character flaws of our forebears can be an impetus toward avoiding certain pitfalls in life, such as addictive behaviours. We predict that those whose family history research is intensely motivated by the quest for self-discovery are likely to be those who are less secure in their sense of self and, thus, more likely to demonstrate lower levels of emotional stability than those less motivated by identity concerns. Possible reasons include that they are missing some crucial information about family (for example the identity of a parent or grandparent) or that they have made discoveries or experienced events that shake their sense of self, such as migrating to a new country, a relationship breakdown or the uncovering of a distasteful family secret.

On a different note, there is also research suggesting that many family historians see themselves as 'kin keepers', inspired by wanting to acknowledge and honour their ancestors by passing on their stories to a new generation, often with the goal of strengthening family feeling and family ties (Bishop 2005; Chance 1988; Kramer 2011b; Walters 2020) or 'leaving a legacy' to one's descendants that helps new generations to understand themselves. Both Erikson (1980) and McAdams (2001) theorise the importance for older adults of establishing a sense of generativity, by which they mean making a contribution toward the next generation through nurturing and mentoring of young people and/or providing some kind of legacy for future generations. It has been argued that family history research is a way of fulfilling this drive toward generativity, in that by passing down their stories, people experience the satisfaction of knowing they are contributing to the lives of those who will succeed them (Hadis 2002).

Indeed, research has shown that intergenerational narratives shared within families are positively related to well-being among adolescent children (Duke et al. 2003, 2008; Merrill and Fivush 2016) and also to stronger family bonding, satisfaction and functioning (Koenig Kellas 2007). It is feasible that the desire to share their stories with family may be more evident among family historians who have developed a stronger sense of generativity, as well as among those who have children and grandchildren with whom they share a common ancestry.

A third psychosocial motive that has been postulated for intense interest in family history research is the cognitive challenge of a complex puzzle to be solved, one that requires new learning, organisation and persistence. A few studies suggest that the detective work of the genealogical research process becomes, for some, an end in itself, with genealogists often reporting elation and other strong emotions as they discover a new link or break down a 'brick wall' (Bishop 2008; Darby and Clough 2013; Hershkovitz and Hardof-Jaffe 2017). Shaw (2020), in a large-scale study of the motives of Australian family historians, described the largest group of her sample (44%) as 'seekers' who were trying to solve a mystery or puzzle associated with their heritage. Additionally, curiosity and love of history were key motivators of a further 16%. An expectation regarding this cognitive challenge motive is that it is likely to be stronger among those with higher educational levels.

The current research was designed to describe the psychosocial motives driving amateur family historians and to pilot an internally reliable measure of the strength of these motives. The construct validity of the measure was examined through factor analysis and correlations with demographic and personality variables. It was postulated that a valid measure of motivational strength would correlate with time spent doing family history research and the perceived importance attributed to this leisure activity, and that motivational factors would show meaningful relationships with personality and demographic data.

The study focusses on non-professional (i.e., amateur) family historians, because this is a group who participate in genealogy research for motives other than to earn a living. Studying this group means that there is less likelihood of conflating psychosocial motives with working life constraints.

A measure of psychosocial motives for and strength of participation in family history research has the potential to be useful as a counselling tool. For example, clients can be made aware that their family history research might assist—or present possible setbacks—to managing and achieving life and relationship goals, such as healing broken relationships, coming to terms with past trauma, or finding life meaning (e.g., Bohanek et al. 2006; Champagne 1990; Green 2013; Merrill and Fivush 2016). Getting counselling clients to focus on their family history through the use of a motive measure can be a stimulus for life review (e.g., Bhar 2017) or point the way to processes for dealing with grief following the death of a loved one (e.g., Darongkamas and Lorenc 2008). Additionally, it can stimulate analysis of how negative behaviour patterns of ancestors can be repeated through generations—an insight that can assist in breaking maladaptive patterns such as domestic violence or addiction (e.g., Allen 2013). The motive measure may also be useful for educational planning, such as assessing student interests, or for marketing of genealogical products and further research.

2. Materials and Methods

2.1. Participants

The selection criteria for participants were that they must be Australian citizens or residents, 18 years or over, and engaged in family history research as a leisure pursuit (rather than a profession). Data from those who did not meet the selection criteria or who did not complete the Motivations Scale (see Method) were not included in analysis. Eligible surveys were completed by 775 adult Australian men and women who self-described as amateur family historians. They were aged between 21 and 93 years, with a median age of 63 years. The majority ($N = 657$; 85%) were women, probably a reasonably accurate reflection of the gender balance in this area. All states of Australia were represented, with the majority from the most populous states, Victoria (35.5%) and NSW (30.1%). Given the predominance of older age groups, it is not surprising that just over half lived with a partner only (51.5%), 18.0% lived alone, and just 18.8% still had children living at home (the remainder were in a variety of different living situations).

Most participants were married or in a long-term relationship (71.8%), 11.5% were single, 11.1% were divorced or separated, and 5.6% were widowed. Most were born in Australia (91.7%) or the UK (5.7%), limiting the possibility of cross-cultural comparisons within this study. They were a highly educated group, with 53.5% having completed a university degree or post-graduate studies. Just over 80% had at least one child, and 50.4% had at least one grandchild. Most (88.3%) had at least one sibling, and 14.1% had one or more half-siblings. Interestingly, 22 people in the sample (2.8%) self-identified as adopted or conceived via donor egg or sperm.

The average amount of time participants spent per week on family history research varied widely from between 5 h or fewer (35.7%), to 6–10 h (27.5%), 11–20 h (19.8%), and more than 20 h (17.1%). When asked to compare the perceived importance of their family history activity to other leisure activities, only 4.2% viewed it as less important, 36.3% as 'about the same', 35.4% as more important, and 24.1% as much more important.

2.2. Ethics

Ethics approval of the project was obtained in July 2018 from the Human Research Ethics Committee of the first author's university, following our submission of materials showing how informed consent, privacy, and confidentiality would be assured (detailed information statement to all participants, anonymous survey, potentially identifying information removed from any published quotes). Non-coercive recruitment processes were used, such that participants had to 'opt in' to complete the survey after viewing an advertisement, Facebook post, or general email from their family history or other interest group. Permission was given for the survey to be conducted in Australia only, given that other countries may have different legislation, regulations, permissions, and customs associated with data collection online. Data collection from other countries would require overseas contact persons to negotiate these constraints, and this was considered beyond the scope of our pilot project.

2.3. Recruitment

An online survey was set up using Qualtrics software. We contacted major genealogical societies throughout Australia, describing the project and asking them to share the survey link. We also placed a brief description of the project and the survey link on several Facebook pages dedicated to family history and DNA research. Additionally, the survey link was shared with students in the University of Tasmania's Diploma of Family History course and on the Australian Psychological Society's members website. The survey remained open for six weeks. The selection criteria were: aged 18 years or older; currently live in Australia; self-describe as 'amateur family historian' (defined as engaging in family history research in an unpaid or mostly unpaid capacity).

2.4. Measures

The following measures relevant to the current analysis were part of a longer online survey of family historian characteristics.

2.5. Psychosocial Motivations for Family History Research (Motivation Scale)

We designed a list of possible motives for engaging in family history research by examining motives suggested in the current literature, and brainstorming items associated with these motives. The list of items was piloted by asking several active family historian researchers to comment and make suggestions about content and format. Feedback was incorporated into a final scale of 20 items, this number considered as being of manageable length while adequately covering a range of content. The scale was designed to measure the strength of motivation to research family history, in general and potentially across different motivational categories.

Participants were given the following instructions: "Below are some reasons that people participate in family history research. Please rate the importance of these reasons for you, in the table below". The rating scale comprised 'very important' (scored 2), 'somewhat important' (scored 1), or 'not important' (scored 0). Item 20, 'other reasons' was not scored, but if participants checked this as either somewhat or very important, they were asked to list these reasons. This open-ended option provided the opportunity for us to collect qualitative data and to potentially develop the scale for future research, in an area where previous research has been limited. The scale used is presented in full in Table 1.

Table 1. Per cent responses to reasons for participating in family history ($N = 775$).

	I Participate in Family History Research:	Very Important %	Somewhat Important %	Not Important %
1	It's intellectually stimulating	59.1	33.5	7.4
2	To meet like-minded people	13.3	48.4	38.3
3	To give something to my family	49.3	42.1	8.6
4	To bring my family together	17.0	48.4	34.6
5	To make a contribution to future generations	58.8	34.1	7.1
6	To acknowledge those who came before me	75.0	20.9	4.1
7	To find out more about who I am	61.7	30.3	8.0
8	To improve my self-esteem and sense of worth	7.0	27.2	65.8
9	To discover why I am like I am	16.8	47.5	35.7
10	To find out more about my ethnic background	33.3	44.8	21.9

Table 1. Cont.

	I Participate in Family History Research:	Very Important %	Somewhat Important %	Not Important %
11	Curiosity about my roots	76.3	22.5	1.3
12	It is something to talk about to others	10.1	48.4	41.5
13	It keeps my mind active	57.9	34.1	8.0
14	To find out more about my health history and risk factors	9.9	34.8	55.2
15	To solve a family mystery or prove a family story	39.7	33.5	26.7
16	To find a lost relative	25.2	32.4	42.5
17	To become a professional family historian	9.9	21.4	68.6
18	To use my talents and skills	43.7	41.3	15.0
19	Because I love history	68.0	24.8	7.2
20	Other reasons (if you have other reasons please list them below)	12.3	8.8	79.0

2.6. Demographic Data

Participants were asked to respond to survey items concerning their age, gender, educational and relationship status, family characteristics, living situation, country of birth, whether they were adopted or donor-conceived, whether they had undertaken a DNA test, number of hours per week spent researching family history, and the perceived importance of their family history research in relation to other leisure activities.

2.7. Personality

Two measures of personality were used: the first to obtain a broad picture of the strength of major personality characteristics among this sample of family historian researchers and the second to target the extent to which different motives for conducting family history research relate to generativity, a developmental characteristic associated with the desire to provide for younger generations through nurturing, mentoring, and leaving a legacy.

(a) Big Five Personality Inventory (Shortened Version). The 10-item short version of the Big Five Personality Inventory (NEO-PI-R; Costa and McCrae 1992) was used (Rammstedt and John 2007). This scale is designed to measure personality through five factors, which have been described as its key overarching variables, these being extraversion (sociable and outgoing), agreeableness (compliant, trusting, and warm), conscientiousness (organised and strong work ethic), neuroticism (anxious, opposite to emotional stability) and openness (enjoys new experiences, creative, and nonjudgmental) (Costa and McCrae 1992). The shortened scale has two items each for each factor and has demonstrated adequate reliability and validity across several studies (Rammstedt 2007; Rammstedt et al. 2020; Rammstedt and John 2007). Respondents are asked to self-describe (I see myself as someone who is . . .) in relation to 10 words or phrases (e.g., relaxed; gets nervous easily). There are five response options ranging from disagree strongly (1) to agree strongly (5). One item is reversed for each personality factor.

(b) Generativity. The generativity scale is an eight-item scale based on Erikson's description of generativity as an individual's perception that they have engaged in activities that nurture the next generation or create things that will outlast them (Moore and Rosenthal 2014). Items are designed to cover the range of general life domains in which one can make a contribution, as well as an individual's overview of the extent to which they assess their life as worthwhile and productive (e.g., "So far my life has been worthwhile; I have made a contribution to society through my family"). Responses can range from strongly disagree (1) to strongly agree (5). Items are summed to form a generativity scale with a possible range of 8–40. The scale shows high alpha reliability in the current study (0.86) and there is evidence of strong alpha reliability and construct validity from a previous study (Moore and Rosenthal 2014).

2.8. Analyses

The motives items were factor analysed. Scales were developed for the total measure of motive strength and the subscale factors. These scales/subscales were assessed for internal reliability and construct validity. The qualitative data derived from the 'other' response was examined to ascertain whether respondents identified motives not assessed in our pilot scale.

3. Results

Table 1 shows the per cent response to each item on the Motivation Scale. Curiosity (item 11), love of history (item 15), acknowledging ancestors (item 6), and 'finding out more about who I am' (item 7) were the most popular reasons given for participating in family history. Most items were rated as somewhat or very important by more than half the participants, the exceptions being item 8 (improving self-esteem), item 14 (finding out about health risks), and item 17 (becoming a professional family historian).

The 19 items were subjected to a Principal Components factor analysis with Varimax Rotation. The Scree test suggested that a three-factor solution most economically and meaningfully grouped the data. Three items with cross loadings were removed (Items 2, 8, and 12). The remaining 16 items were re-analysed and produced three distinct factors (shown with factor loadings in Table 2), which together accounted for 46.23% of the variance of the items.

Table 2. Rotated component matrix for factor analysis of the Psychosocial Motivations for Family History Research Scale.

	Factor 1	Factor 2	Factor 3
To find out more about my ethnic background	0.675		
To find a lost relative	0.664		
To solve a family mystery/disprove a family story	0.641		
To discover reasons why I am like I am	0.626		
To find out more about health history/risk factors	0.569		
To find out more about who I am	0.547		
Curiosity about my roots	0.472		
To give something to my family		0.809	
To make a contribution to future generations		0.782	
To bring my family together		0.712	
To acknowledge who came before me		0.612	
To use my talents and skills			0.778
It keeps my mind active			0.727
Because it is intellectually stimulating			0.715
Because I love history			0.536
To become a professional family historian			0.452

Factor 1 (17.39% of the rotated variance) comprised seven items relating to being motivated by the desire to find out more about oneself and one's ancestral/cultural influences. It was labelled *Self-Understanding Motive*. Factor 2 (14.94% of the variance) consisted of four items relating to altruistic motives for engaging in family history, for example the desire to contribute to future generations. It was labelled *Altruism Motive*. Factor 3 (five items, 13.90% of the variance) concerned the intellectual challenges of family history research, for example keeping the mind active. This factor was labelled *Cognitive Challenge*.

Scales were formed by adding the ratings of items that made up the factors. The Self-Understanding Motive scale comprised items 7, 9, 11, 14, 15, and 16. The Altruism Motive scale comprised items 3, 4, 5, and 6, and the Cognitive Challenge scale comprised items 1, 3, 17, 18, and 19. The Total Motivation scale was the sum of all items except 2, 8, and 12, which were removed from the final version because of their cross loadings.

Table 3 shows the means, standard deviations, possible ranges, and alpha reliability coefficients of the total scale and the subscales. Reliabilities were considered adequate for research purposes, although the alpha for Cognitive Challenge is a little low. Conventionally, in test development, an alpha level of 0.7 and above is considered satisfactory, while 0.8 and above is considered high; however, a range of qualitative descriptors has been used for this index. Several writers have described alphas of 0.6 to 0.69 as 'adequate' or 'acceptable', the implication being that a higher level of the index would increase trust (Taber 2018). Alphas were not improved by the removal of items.

Table 3. Motive Scale Statistics.

	No. Items	Mean	SD	Possible Range	Alpha
Motive Strength (total scale)	16	19.50	5.31	0–32	0.80
Factor 1 Self Understanding Motive	7	7.71	3.03	0–14	0.74
Factor 2 Altruism Motive	4	5.46	1.91	0–8	0.76
Factor 3 Cognitive Challenge Motive	5	6.33	2.17	0–10	0.68

Intercorrelations between subscales were as follows: Self-Understanding and Altruism, 0.42; Self-Understanding and Cognitive Challenge, 0.28; Altruism and Cognitive Challenge, 0.25. These moderate intercorrelations indicate that while the subscales were somewhat related, they are also relatively independent.

Construct Validity

Table 4 shows correlations between the motive scales and several demographic and personality variables.

Table 4. Correlations between factors, demographic and personality variables.

Factors	Strength Motive	Self Understanding Motive	Altruism Motive	Cognitive Challenge Motive
Age	−0.13 *	−0.12 *	−0.02	−0.13 *
Gender (1 = M, 2 = F)	0.14 *	0.15 *	0.06	0.08
Education	−0.06	−0.14 *	−0.09	0.12 *
No. children	0.07	0.05	0.15 *	−0.03
No. grandchildren	0.04	0.04	0.10 *	−0.04
Half-sibs?	0.07	0.15 *	0.01	−0.05
Adopted?	0.06	0.12 *	0.02	−0.03
Importance of FH	24 *	0.13 *	0.17 *	0.26 *
Hrs/week on FH	0.06	0.00	0.03	0.11 *
DNA test?	0.07	0.11 *	0.02	0.01
Generativity	0.21 *	0.09	0.24 *	0.18 *
Extraversion	0.05	0.06	0.08	−0.04
Agreeableness	−0.02	−0.05	0.05	0.00
Conscientiousness	0.12 *	0.05	0.14 *	0.10 *
Emotional stability	−0.08	−0.11 *	−0.03	−0.03
Openness	0.10 *	0.08	0.11 *	0.05

Notes: * $p < 0.01$; FH = family history.

With respect to the total scale, those who expressed stronger motives to research family history were significantly younger (within an older population), more likely to be female, and to rate their family history hobby as relatively more important than other leisure activities. Interestingly, however, time spent on family history did not correlate with total motivational strength, only to the Cognitive Challenge subscale. In terms of personality and developmental stage, greater motive strength was associated with higher levels of conscientiousness, openness, and generativity.

With respect to the subscales, those who scored higher on any of the three motivational factors were also more likely to rate their family history hobby as relatively more important than their other leisure pursuits. On other variables, however, the profiles differed.

Those with stronger motives to search for self-understanding were also younger and less educated than the sample as a whole. They were more likely to be female, have half-siblings, be adopted or donor-conceived, have taken a genealogical DNA test, and be somewhat less emotionally stable than the rest of the sample.

Those characterised by stronger altruistic motives for their family history research did not differ from the rest of the sample on age, gender, or education but they were likely to have more children and grandchildren than those with weaker altruistic motives. High altruism was associated with a stronger sense of generativity plus greater conscientious and openness to experience.

Finally, those more strongly motivated by the cognitive challenges of family history research were younger, better educated, and spent more time on their genealogical hobby than those with lower levels of this motive. These 'genealogical detectives' were characterised by high generativity and conscientiousness.

Twenty-one per cent of the sample rated 'other' motives as very or somewhat important as drivers of their family history research, resulting in 163 (mostly very brief) descriptions of such motives. The initial stimulus for taking an interest in family history was frequently mentioned. People said they were challenged to engage in family history research after events such as "when my father died", "because my daughter had a school project", or "after I inherited a box full of old family photos". We chose not to categorise these stimuli as psychosocial motives; although they may account for getting started, they do not explain persistence with the hobby.

Most of the remaining responses were a restatement of one of the three motives already described, or a combination of these, sometimes with specific family examples or stories attached. For example, different aspects of self-understanding were mentioned, including personal, cultural, and biological identity (respectively), as shown in the quotes below (responding to the stem, I participate in family history research):

To really try to understand my place in the world

I am Aboriginal so it is important to discover and uncover those who were taken from us, understand our huge mob and extensive family connections.

I am an adoptee and wanted to find out who my father and mother were and also to find out about my biological parents' background and where they came from.

Altruistic motives were also commonly mentioned, for example:

It gives me a buzz when I find a relative, or when helping others with their research—i.e., brick walls. I love it when I can break down a brick wall for someone, it gives them great pleasure and me also.

I am simply interested in where we came from and would like to pass that information on to future generations in our family.

I want, in at least some small way, to honour those who went before me by telling their stories.

Thirdly, the cognitive challenge motive was reiterated frequently, for example:

I enjoy the challenge.

I love the intellectual challenge of family research, the insights I gain into ancestors' lives in their country of origin and in Australia, and the historical context in which they lived.

I love a mystery and want to solve as many family mysteries as I can. I am very curious and want to satisfy that in me.

A combination of the three motives occurred in some responses:

I am an only child and feel that family trees encourage me to understand my family's lives. I also love the chase, the problem-solving part gives me a pat on the back that once I retired, wasn't there anymore. But my strongest reason is that I love my family, I knew two great grandmothers, and it shows me a young person was there inside all the time. I'm seeing and understanding this now.

Were any new reasons for participating in family history research revealed? A few respondents gave examples of motives that we had not included in our measure. We isolated four different reasons, each of which was mentioned by more than one person (but fewer than 10). The reasons were:

(a) Spiritual or life-meaning motives. These responses mentioned a specific religion, or some spiritual or transcendental reason for engaging in family history research. For example:

My paternal grandmother read tea leaves and tarot cards and my maternal grandmother could intuit future events. Both my parents were Spiritualists able to "see" and "hear" messages from beyond the veil. My oldest daughter is now a professional psychic. Those of us in our family who follow this tradition believe we have an ongoing connection to those ancestors who have passed on and it stimulates our interest in their lives.

I'm getting older, and family history is part of my wondering about why are we all here/what's life all about?

I went to a clairvoyant and she talked about my family members that had passed over. I wanted to know something about them and 22 years later still finding out information.

I am a Latter-Day Saint and it is important to us to know our ancestry.

(b) Comfort motives. Comfort was viewed as a motive for family history participation by several people. These feelings seemed to go beyond the relaxation that is generally provided by hobbies and included relief from strong negative emotions, such as those associated with serious illness and grief. For example:

It is a major stress relieving hobby—you have to concentrate to do it well so you forget other life pressures.

I am terminally ill although I wasn't when I started. I find it gives me comfort.

I have lived with chronic illness for 33 years. It has been a life saver when times are tough. I can focus on research and forget about problems.

My father passed away suddenly then three close relatives also died within six weeks. I didn't want to answer the phone anymore. But this is when I started looking for deceased people [in the family tree]. It helped me come to terms with the loss of my father.

(c) Making social connections. Another motive for persisting with family history research was the enjoyment of the social connections made. We had included two items relating to social connections in the initial measure, but they did not form a clear factor. Inclusion of more items tapping this concept may be advisable, given that there were several different aspects of social connection mentioned, including getting to know other amateur family historians, becoming more engaged with the professional genealogical community, and meeting previously unknown relatives. Examples include being motivated to engage in family history because:

I enjoy being part of the genealogical community.

For social purposes: giving an infrastructure or reason for meeting and interacting with distant relations.

I attend local, state, national and international conferences now and meet a wide range of likeminded people. It gives me more opportunity to make connections that weren't around when I started.

(d) Travel enhancement. Finally, several people commented on how their family history research enhanced their travel experiences and perceived this as a motive for continuing their research. For example:

> It makes travel more interesting by merging historical context into places you travel and if you specifically travel for family history it brings alive the context of past times (and can make our modern life pressures seem trivial in comparison to the barriers faced by ancestors).

> [It's] a reason to travel. For geographical and nature study reasons: exploring beautifully placed old cemeteries with their own wild gardens in far flung places. For a sense of belonging in a place: to be driving through a town or even a street and noting that that's where a certain relative lived or be driving past a cemetery where another relative is buried.

> I have travelled all over Britain to where my ancestors come from and walked the streets they walked, stayed on the islands they lived on, walked the graveyards, visited the churches, and enriched my travels in the process. And now I'm "hooked"!

4. Discussion

In this study, three psychosocial motives for engaging in family history research were described and assessed, and scales were developed to measure their strength. The motives were conceptualised as relating to underlying and relatively persistent psychological processes rather than to initiating events that led to short-term interest only, for example the need to write a eulogy or help a child with a school assignment (although events of this type may also trigger longer-term engagement with genealogical research). The measure of motive strength and its factorially obtained subscales of motive strength in specific areas (Self-Understanding Motive, Altruism Motive, and Cognitive Challenge) all showed adequate Cronbach alpha reliabilities, although piloting with additional items might be worthwhile to strengthen these reliabilities further, particularly for Cognitive Challenge.

The total scale and the subscales also showed evidence of construct validity. As might be expected, higher scores on each of the four measures related to greater perceived importance of participants' family history engagement in comparison with their other hobbies and interests. Additionally, the subscales demonstrated differing patterns of association with demographic and personality variables that were consistent with the different motivational constructs we were aiming to measure, as described below.

Individuals whose motives toward self-understanding were stronger were also more likely to be adopted, have half-siblings, and/or have had a DNA test. These associations independently suggest a lack of knowledge about biological and ancestral roots (for example, possibly unknown biological parents or grandparents). The finding of lower levels of emotional stability among those with higher scores on the self-understanding motive fits with the notion that there may be some distress associated with lack of knowledge about one's ancestral and cultural background. The lack of knowledge may point to feelings of not belonging and of not being sure of one's place in the world, and even a weakened sense of identity.

Higher scores on the altruism motive were characteristic of those who had more descendants and who were more generative, that is, oriented toward assisting and leaving a legacy for the next generation. The higher levels of conscientiousness and openness to experience of these individuals also points to a sense of personal maturity that might reasonably characterise those with the psychosocial resources to contribute toward the welfare of others, particularly with activities that strengthen family ties.

Finally, those more strongly motivated by the cognitive challenges of family history research tended to be more highly educated and to spend more time on their genealogical activities; this pattern of associations is consistent with the motivational construct we were attempting to measure with the Cognitive Challenge subscale. It indicates an interest in intellectual endeavours, puzzles and mysteries, and the at-times addictive quality of these interests.

The question arises as to whether the three motives we delineated and measured are adequate to describe the major psychosocial motivating forces behind strong engagement with family history. Certainly, each of the scale items was viewed by survey participants as an important or very important reason for participating in their hobby, which for the majority of the sample was viewed as more important than their other leisure pursuits. Given the opportunity to indicate other major motives, study participants mostly redescribed those motives we had already assessed, or indicated an initial stimulus for beginning their genealogical research rather than a motive for continued engagement. Only a small number of people described motives for their genealogical research that were different from our initial conceptualisations.

However, it may be of value in further research to expand our pilot measure through the inclusion of items that could form subscales to assess the four additional motives described in the qualitative data: spiritual/life meaning motives, comfort motives, making social connections, and travel enhancement. With respect to social connections, we had included two items relating to this motive/reason in the original measure, but they did not form a clear factor (nor were they assessed as very important overall). As mentioned previously, several more social connection items could be added to our scale in order to tap various aspects of this concept. Items could include the desire to meet previously unknown relatives, make new friendships, join groups with like-minded interests and engage in professional networking. Social connection is a motive underlying many if not most leisure activities. Unless one is seeking a specific living relative, it may not seem an obvious stimulus for starting out genealogical research, but the plethora of interest and support groups in this area suggest it may provide a motive to persist.

As well as for social connections, items assessing spiritual/religious, comfort/stress relief, and travel enhancement motives could be developed through attention to the qualitative research described above, along with brainstorming or further surveying of family historians. Using a new participant sample, rating and factor analysis of a new, longer scale of around 50 or more items could assess the viability of the original factors and the existence of new ones. The comfort motive is particularly interesting from the point of view of more widely incorporating family history discussion and research into counselling practice. The potential of genealogy to assist individuals in dealing with trauma, grief, and life transitions has been recognised in the literature (e.g., Champagne 1990; Darongkamas and Lorenc 2008) and has also been noted by some of our research participants. Development of this aspect of a revised motives scale could both highlight and assess to what extent family history research contributes to mental health outcomes, especially among older individuals, for whom the value of life review and reminiscence has been demonstrated (Bhar 2017).

Our study is limited in so far as our sample, while large, comprised Australian residents only, most of them from older age groups. Additionally, the multiculturalism of Australian society was not reflected in the sample, with almost all participants having been born in Australia. We did not examine cultural background in a more general way, for example through assessing religion, perceived ethnicity, or parents' and grandparents' countries of birth, nor were we able able to compare Australian data with that from other countries. We did not examine (or ask about) race or indigenous background. These limitations are important because genetic connections ("blood ties") may not be as significant to feelings of identity and belongingness in some cultures as they are in others, for example in cultures where parenting duties are shared across a tribe, clan, or neighbourhood, or cultures where identity is as much tied to place as it is to parentage. Further, the honouring of ancestors may play a more important role in strongly religious cultures than it does in those that are more secular, given that most religions emphasise respect for one's forebears. Examples include the fourth commandment of the Judeo-Christian religions and the filial piety and obedience expectations of Confucianism. Further research could, for example, examine popularity and motivation to conduct family history research among cultures differing on dimensions such as religiosity, individualism/collectivism, and parenting styles, as well as among younger age groups.

Despite these limitations, we believe our scale provides a starting point for further study of the intensity and differentiation of motives to research one's ancestry, and to examine how these motives relate to characteristics of the researcher and to the range of both positive and negative psychosocial outcomes they derive from their searches. To date, we know little about genealogy as a leisure pursuit and how it compares to other hobbies in terms of its contribution to self-understanding and mental health. It is hoped that the measure we have piloted will be of use to other researchers who wish to build on the recent work of Moore et al. (2021), Shaw (2020), and Walters (2020) in examining the psychology underpinning this popular pastime.

Author Contributions: The authors contributed equally to the conceptualisation of this paper. Both authors have read and agreed to the published version of the manuscript.

Funding: This research received no external funding.

Institutional Review Board Statement: The study was conducted according to the guidelines of the Declaration of Helsinki, and approved by the Swinburne University of Technology Human Research Ethics Committee (protocol code 2018/242; date of approval: 19 July 2018).

Informed Consent Statement: Informed consent was obtained from all subjects involved in the study.

Data Availability Statement: Queries about data can be directed to Emeritus Professor Susan Moore, e-mail: smoore@swin.edu.au.

Acknowledgments: We thank those genealogical organisations who assisted us in recruiting study participants and the Australian Psychological Society and the University of Tasmania Diploma of Family History staff who posted links to the study on their websites. We also thank the study participants for their thoughtful contributions, and research assistant Alex Poll who helped us set up the survey on Qualtrics and in many other ways.

Conflicts of Interest: The authors declare no conflict of interest.

References

Allen, David M. 2013. The Historical Backdrop of Family Dysfunction. Family Dysfunction and Mental Health Blog. Available online: http://davidmallenmd.blogspot.com/2013/06/the-historical-backdrop-of-family.html (accessed on 8 August 2021).
Bhar, Sunil. 2017. Reminiscence therapy. In *The SAGE Encyclopedia of Abnormal and Clinical Psychology*. Edited by A. Wenzel. Thousand Oaks: SAGE Publications, Inc, pp. 2848–49.
Birt, Linda, Jon D. Emery, A. Toby Prevost, Stephen Sutton, and Fiona M. Walter. 2014. Psychological impact of family history risk assessment in primary care: A mixed methods study. *Family Practice* 31: 409–18. [CrossRef]
Bishop, Ronald. 2005. "The essential force of the clan": Developing a collecting-inspired ideology of genealogy through textual analysis. *Journal of Popular Culture* 38: 990–1010. [CrossRef]
Bishop, Ronald. 2008. In the grand scheme of things: An exploration of the meaning of genealogical research. *Journal of Popular Culture* 41: 393–412. [CrossRef]
Bohanek, Jennifer, Kelly Marin, Robyn Fivush, and Marshall Duke. 2006. Family narrative interaction and children's sense of self. *Family Process* 45: 39–54. [CrossRef]
Bottero, Wendy. 2012. Who do you think they were? How family historians make sense of social position and inequality in the past. *British Journal of Sociology* 63: 54–74. [CrossRef]
Bottero, Wendy. 2015. Practising family history: 'Identity' as a category of social practice. *British Journal of Sociology* 66: 534–56. [CrossRef] [PubMed]
Champagne, Delight E. 1990. The genealogical search as a counseling technique. *Journal of Counseling & Development* 69: 85–87.
Chance, Sue. 1988. The psychological functions of genealogy in the aged. *Journal of Geriatric Psychiatry and Neurology* 1: 113–15. [CrossRef] [PubMed]
Costa, Paul T., and Robert R. McCrae. 1992. *NEO-PI-R Professional Manual*. Odessa: Psychological Assessment Resources.
Darby, Paul, and Paul Clough. 2013. Investigating the information-seeking behaviour of genealogists and family historians. *Journal of Information Science* 39: 73–84. [CrossRef]
Darongkamas, Jurai, and Louise Lorenc. 2008. Going back to our roots. *Psychologist* 21: 1022–25.
Duke, Marshall, Robyn Fivush, Amber Lazarus, and Jennifer Bohanek. 2003. *Of Ketchup and Kin: Dinnertime Conversations as a Major Source of Family Knowledge, Family Adjustment, and Family Resilience (Working Paper 027–03)*. Atlanta: Center for the Study of Myth and Ritual in American Life, Emory University.
Duke, Marshall, Amber Lazarus, and Robyn Fivush. 2008. Knowledge of family history as a clinically useful index of psychological well-being and prognosis: A brief report. *Psychotherapy* 45: 268–72. [CrossRef] [PubMed]
Erikson, Erik. 1980. *Identity and the Life Cycle*. New York: W.W. Norton and Co.
Green, Anna. 2013. Intergenerational family stories: Private, parochial, pathological? *Journal of Family History* 38: 387–402. [CrossRef]

Hadis, Martin. 2002. From Generation to Generation: Family Stories, Computers and Genealogy. Master thesis, Media Arts and Sciences, Massachusetts Institute of Technology, Cambridge, MA, USA. Available online: http://citeseerx.ist.psu.edu/viewdoc/download?doi=10.1.1.475.5115&rep=rep1&type=pdf (accessed on 1 June 2021).

Hershkovitz, Arnon, and Sharon Hardof-Jaffe. 2017. Genealogy as a lifelong learning endeavor. *Leisure/Loisir* 41: 535–60. [CrossRef]

Hertz, Joan E. 1998. In pursuit of authenticity: An adoptee's quest. *Modern Psychoanalysis* 23: 103–12.

Koenig Kellas, Jody. 2007. Family ties: Communicating identity through jointly told family stories. *Communication Monographs* 72: 365–89.

Kramer, Anne-Maree. 2011a. Mediatizing memory: History, affect and identity in Who Do You Think You Are? *European Journal of Cultural Studies* 14: 428–45. [CrossRef]

Kramer, Anne-Maree. 2011b. Kinship, affinity and connectedness: Exploring the role of genealogy in personal lives. *Sociology* 45: 379–95. [CrossRef]

Lambert, Ronald D. 1996. The family historian and temporal orientations towards the ancestral past. *Time & Society* 5: 115–43.

McAdams, Dan. 2001. The psychology of life stories. *Review of General Psychology* 5: 100–22. [CrossRef]

Merrill, Natalie, and Robyn Fivush. 2016. Intergenerational narratives and identity across development. *Developmental Review* 40: 72–92. [CrossRef]

Moore, Susan, and Doreen Rosenthal. 2014. Personal growth, grandmother engagement and satisfaction among non-custodial grandmothers. *Ageing and Mental Health* 9: 136–43. [CrossRef] [PubMed]

Moore, Susan, Doreen Rosenthal, and Rebecca Robinson. 2021. *The Psychology of Family History: Exploring Our Genealogy*. Abingdon: Taylor & Francis.

Müller, Ulrich, and Barbara Perry. 2001. Adopted persons' search for and contact with their birth parents I: Who searches and why? *Adoption Quarterly* 4: 5–37. [CrossRef]

Parham, Angel Adams. 2008. Race, memory and family history. *Social Identities* 14: 13–32. [CrossRef]

Rammstedt, Beatrice. 2007. The 10-Item Big Five Inventory: Norm values and investigation of sociodemographic effects based on a German population representative sample. *European Journal of Psychological Assessment* 23: 193–201. [CrossRef]

Rammstedt, Beatrice, and Oliver P. John. 2007. Measuring personality in one minute or less A 10-item short version of the Big Five Inventory in English and German. *Journal of Research in Personality* 41: 203–12. [CrossRef]

Rammstedt, Beatrice, Daniel Danner, Christopher J. Soto, and Oliver P. John. 2020. Validation of the short and extra-short forms of the Big Five Inventory-2 and their German adaptations. *European Journal of Psychological Assessment* 36: 149–61. [CrossRef]

Shaw, Emma. 2020. "Who we are, and why we do it": A demographic overview and the cited motivations of Australia's family historians. *Journal of Family History* 45: 109–24. [CrossRef]

Sobol, Michael P., and Jeanette Cardiff. 1983. A sociopsychological investigation of adult adoptees' search for birth parents. *Family Relations* 32: 477–83. [CrossRef]

Spector, Tim. 2013. How your grandparents' life could have changed your genes. *The Conversation*. Available online: https://theconversation.com/how-your-grandparents-life-could-have-changed-your-genes-19136 (accessed on 1 June 2021).

Taber, Keith S. 2018. The use of Cronbach's Alpha when developing and reporting research instruments in Science Education. *Research in Science Education* 48: 1273–96. [CrossRef]

Walters, Penny. 2020. *The Psychology of Searching*. London: Author.

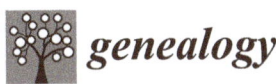

Article

Pilgrimage and Purpose: Ancestor Research as Sacred Practice in a Secular Age

Rebecca Robinson

Faculty of Information Technology, Monash University, Melbourne 3800, Australia; rebecca.robinson@monash.edu

Abstract: This paper explores the ways in which ancestor research has become a replacement for religious community and practice in a post-religious world. We explore the parallels of popular present-day family history pursuits with traditional religious practices, noting the similarities in how the practices are used to foster and strengthen feelings of identity, purpose, and belonging. We look at three particular customs that are common to those interested in ancestor research: the handing on of 'sacred' stories and objects with familial significance; acts of pilgrimage to ancestrally significant places; and engaging in 'ritual' gatherings, either with extended family or with others who share the interest of ancestor research.

Keywords: secular rituals; post-religious; sacred stories; pilgrimage; family ritual; ceremony

1. Introduction

For Western, English-speaking countries such as the US, UK, and Australia, the practice of religion—Christianity in particular—was long taken for granted as central to the culture and to public life. Going to church on Sunday was once something most families simply did each week, and to stray from this cultural norm would make one stand out in the community. However, since the latter half of the twentieth century, the religious landscape has changed drastically in these Christian-majority countries. To some extent, this has been a result of wider immigration and a broader acceptance of other religious traditions. Furthermore, much has also been made of the rise of what has been termed the "nones and dones"—people who do not attend church or identify with religion of any kind.[1] A recent report by the American-based think tank Pew Research Center (2019, p. 568) describes the religious landscape in the US as changing rapidly, with the percentage of adults describing themselves as Christian dropping from 77% in 2009 down to 65% in 2018–2019. Those identifying as non-religious (atheist, agnostic, or "nothing in particular") have risen from 17% in 2009 up to 26%. Pew Research Center comments specifically on the striking growth of adults in this category over the past thirty years, noting that the University of Chicago's first General Social Survey in 1972 reported only around 5% of adults as non-religious.

In Australia, from the time of British settlement up until the 1950s, the influence of the Christian church wove its way into the fabric of the culture, influencing politics, education systems, morality, and social customs, with the Billy Graham crusades of 1959 giving that decade a particularly strong emphasis on evangelical Christianity. Up until this time, professing atheism or agnosticism would have been seen as highly unusual in Australian society. In the nineteenth century, it was common to assume that "an inability or a refusal to believe in God was a form of mental illness" (Frame 2009, p. 395), and even in the early half of the twentieth century, "anyone who refused to profess religious belief was consciously standing apart from society and popular culture" (p. 91). From the 1960s onwards, however, Australia began its transformation into what some have termed a post-Christian society. By the 1970s, Carey (1996) tells us that "nominal belief coupled with a secular lifestyle" (p. 176) had become a far more acceptable option in Australian society. Census results in

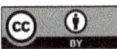

Citation: Robinson, Rebecca. 2021. Pilgrimage and Purpose: Ancestor Research as Sacred Practice in a Secular Age. *Genealogy* 5: 90. https://doi.org/10.3390/genealogy5040090

Received: 19 August 2021
Accepted: 18 October 2021
Published: 21 October 2021

Publisher's Note: MDPI stays neutral with regard to jurisdictional claims in published maps and institutional affiliations.

Copyright: © 2021 by the author. Licensee MDPI, Basel, Switzerland. This article is an open access article distributed under the terms and conditions of the Creative Commons Attribution (CC BY) license (https://creativecommons.org/licenses/by/4.0/).

1971 showed for the first time an increase in the number of people declaring themselves to have no religion (p. 174). In 1991, the census layout was changed to add a "No religion" box for respondents to mark, rather than having to explicitly write "none" (Frame 2009, p. 142) and Carey notes that, by this time, "the combined forces of the two categories 'no religion' and 'no reply' were almost a quarter of the entire population" (p. 174).[2] Carey describes this progression as marking the beginning of a new era, noting that in the past "the decision to stop church attendance, choose a civil rather than a church wedding, or declare a state of unbelief was a major life decision. At the very least it involved a family confrontation" (p. 176). However, the Church no longer retains the level of control it once did over what Frame calls "transcendent experiences" (p. 120). Australians' official beliefs, says Frame, are "essentially humanist" (p. 104).

Such a trajectory is not unique to Australia, with much of Western society having undergone a similar shift over the past century. Canadian philosopher Taylor (2007) describes this change as being from "a condition in which belief was the default option" (p. 12) to one in which unbelief is considered far more acceptable, and in many contexts even assumed as standard. Not long ago, it was accepted without question that the church would in some way be involved in the major events in a person's life—birth, marriage, death—performing sacred rituals (christenings, baptisms, weddings, funerals, last rites) to mark such events, but also maintaining official records and registers of births, deaths, and marriages. Typically, religious officials would create these records and they would be recognised by the state as official documents. Nowadays governments tend to adopt this role in society, divorcing the rituals somewhat from any sense of sacredness, and leaving them more in the domain of administrators and bureaucrats rather than spiritual leaders.

While religion's role in society may be diminished from what it was, it leaves a notable gap in its place, what Roof (1999) describes as "wholeness-hunger" (p. 62) and Taylor describes as the "search for fullness" (pp. 14, 19)—a longing for something beyond our everyday lives, some activity or condition through which "life is fuller, richer, deeper, more worth while [sic], more admirable, more what it should be" (p. 5). Taylor describes how religion, in times gone by, has been seen as the means by which this sense of fullness is achieved—or, alternatively, granted to us by some force beyond ourselves. Bouma (2006) also argues that, within the Australian context, secular humanism "has not proven as satisfying as many thought it would be," and that instead we are moving towards a more varied approach to spirituality in our culture, "in which the religious and spiritual have moved out from the control of both the state and such formal organisations as the church" (p. xiv). Roof corroborates this observation from the US perspective, noting poll results from 1994 report that while 65% of Americans believed "religion was losing its influence in public life", still almost the same number, 62%, claimed "the influence of religion was increasing in their personal lives" (p. 7).

The search for meaning persists, even in the absence of a common acceptance of formal religious belief and practice. Jenkins (2016) argues that "even when people reject or challenge religious traditions, they are often engaging with symbolic religious worlds as they shape identity and interactions with intimate partners, parents, and children" (p. 220). This is what Dissanayake (1988) refers to as "making special", where rituals, ideas, and artifacts are bestowed with unique value and significance, placing them "in a realm different from the everyday" (p. 92). While many ancient religious rituals and beliefs may no longer be seen as relevant or credible in modern society, Jenkins notes that "religiosity and wider cultural beliefs about kin come together in everyday encounters" (p. 222). We still feel a need for ceremony, community, the infusing of the sacred into our life's rituals—things that church and religion once delivered. With the rise of this secular age, many are finding new ways to search for meaning and fulfilment. Taylor describes this as "the sanctification of ordinary life" (p. 179).

In this paper, we explore how practices adopted by family historians might serve to fill some of the gaps left by the decline of religion. We consider how involvement in family history research might provide a less institutionalised approach to pursuing meaning, belonging, transcendence, and sacred practice, in ways that align with the humanist values of modern secular Western culture. This is not a new idea, with Ashton and Hamilton (2007) asking whether family history might "be a substitute for being in heaven" (p. 32), and Jacobson (1986) suggesting that genealogy might form a "substitute or surrogate" for religious practice, particularly for those with a religious upbringing who rejected formal religion later in life (p. 350). Lambert (2002) has explored the idea within a distinctly Australian context, noting how certain secular shifts within the culture have prompted some to look more deeply into their ancestry, such as a rise in multiculturalism, and a decrease in the stigma associated with finding convict ancestry.

Here, we examine the hypothesis specifically within three contexts: firstly, discussing how shared *stories* of importance to family become like sacred texts handed down, and objects with familial significance take the form of sacred talismans. We then look at sacred *places*, specifically the practice of pilgrimage: engaging in a journey quest, whether literally or metaphorically. While this has always been a practice intertwined with spirituality, now we see it becoming more freely adopted, particularly among those who seek to connect with their ancestors and their geographic origins. Finally, we explore the idea of sacred *gatherings* within a family history context: the significance of ritual family celebrations or commemorations, as well as the way in which the gathering of communities who share an interest in ancestry can, like religious groups, take on caring and mutual support roles.

2. Sacred Stories

Storytelling is an essential part of many religious traditions. In times past, intergenerational stories were woven into religious and spiritual practice in such a way that it was an accepted part of life. Stories were handed down from one generation to the next so that people would continue to have a sense of who they were, where they were from, how they belonged, and what kind of lasting significance their lives had. In the Hebrew Bible, the God of the Israelites is often specifically referenced as being the same God worshipped by their ancestors—the God of Abraham, Isaac, and Jacob,[3] reminding the hearer that their relationship to God is one that sits in the context of history and of the many generations who have come before. In fact, long genealogical listings permeate the pages of many books in the Hebrew Bible, used as sacred texts by Jews and Christians alike, in some cases serving meticulous records of each person's tribal inheritance and perhaps eligibility for priesthood or kingship, in other cases telling a deeper story about a particular person and their heritage.

Sacred stories continue to be a part of many different kinds of religious practice today. The oral tradition of handing down stories through poetry, chanting, song, and other forms, is common across many different cultures, for example:

- During the annual Passover *seder*, Jewish families traditionally gather together around a meal and retell the account of the Exodus, to commemorate their ancestors' release from slavery in Egypt and teach the story to the next generation. As part of the ritual, the youngest child present must ask four questions throughout the ceremony, which prompt the telling of the story. The answers are recited in unison by the other guests.
- Ancient writings continue to be read, spoken, and heard by Christian believers today, both as part of personal spiritual discipline and as part of the liturgy in corporate worship. In certain denominations, a particular pre-appointed passage of Scripture (the *lectionary*) is read and preached on each week in every participating church throughout the world. The individual worshipper—aware that other believers all around the globe are hearing the same readings, perhaps in different languages, but containing the same essential message—thus gains a sense of being one part of a larger body (the "Universal Church"), and of being connected to something greater than themselves. There is the knowledge, too, that these texts have been read again and again by hundreds of generations before the present one. In this sense, the believer becomes a part of something greater not just in space, but also in time—part of a "great cloud of witnesses", as it is poetically expressed in the biblical book of Hebrews.[4]

- Such traditions are not limited only to Western culture. In many parts of sub-Saharan Africa, for instance, there is a strong oral tradition, where after dinner the villagers will congregate around a fire to listen to the storyteller, or *griot*, whose role is both to educate and to entertain. The griot was traditionally a role passed down from one generation to the next (although one could also formally train for the role at griot schools), and would serve as storytellers, musicians, historians, genealogists, and counsellors to kings (Encyclopedia Britannica 2014).

Religious writings use the power of story and of narrative to tell tales of identity, heritage, belonging, and redemption. These are stories that have been handed down from parent to child, over and over again—essentially, these are ancient, long-enduring, intergenerational narratives whose meaning and influence has seen them persist through centuries, even millennia, continuing to build a sense of belonging and kinship in each new generation who receives them. However, with what has been termed the "rise of the nones", an increasing number of people do not feel such an attachment to any particular set of ancient sacred texts. Roof (1999) notes that such "grand narratives, handed down through history with appeals to universal truth" (p. 56) are no longer compelling to many of the younger generation. In part, an increased sense of scepticism and a greater familiarity with other cultural backgrounds has perhaps propelled this generation towards more relativistic and individualistic attitudes regarding spirituality. However, Roof also claims that many younger people are simply not as familiar with traditional religious stories as in previous generations, often having been raised without any connection to a formal religious community. In many cases their experience of church attendance may have been limited to weddings and funerals, giving them relatively few opportunities to hear such stories.

It seems that individual family stories and narratives can, and often do, continue to serve a similar role of building a sense of identity and belonging in much the same way as religious texts. As Shaw (2020) describes, telling family stories provides a way for individuals to explain who they are, both to themselves and to others, fulfilling a common desire to "belong to something larger than their singular 'self', [to be] positioned and represented within the broader narrative of humanity" (p. 110). Smith (2006) recounts her experience of hearing her own family stories passed on in such a way that brought to mind a sense of the sacred (pp. 12–13):

> Listening to the senior women telling stories to younger women about the place we were in, or events that were associated with that place, I thought of the stories that members of my own family had told me, and that I would now pass on to my own children. I realized, too, that the meanings I drew out of those stories, and the uses I had made of them, would of course be different to the meanings, and uses, the generations both before and after me had and would construct.

Smith notes that physical, tangible objects such as family heirlooms could be associated with the stories, for example, special table decorations, ornaments, or artworks that have their own family history. Such objects may not be valuable in monetary terms but are precious within the family, taking on their own spiritual significance because of what they represent historically and ancestrally. Handing down these sacred objects to the next generation thus contributes to a person's sense of generativity, of leaving a legacy that has lasting significance.

A survey conducted by Moore et al. (2021) of amateur family historians revealed that "honouring those from the past" is often a key motivator for genealogical research. Moore et al. comment on the "mystical–almost spiritual–feelings" respondents reported regarding this act of paying tribute to their ancestors by learning their stories and writing them down (p. 55). They discuss how the sense of responsibility family historians often feel to hand these stories down to the next generation can propel their research. Such stories can then serve to establish a strong family narrative, something that Feiler (2013) asserts is an essential ingredient in making families "effective, resilient [and] happy". Referencing work from Dr. Marshall Duke, Feiler reports that children with a "strong intergenerational self" who "know they belong to something bigger than themselves" show higher levels of self-confidence.

Driessnack (2017) talks about the importance of intergenerational narratives in providing an "expanded" sense of self that exists in context within a particular time and space, and in relation to family. She notes that the development of this intergenerational self may provide health benefits and contribute to resilience throughout all stages of life. Driessnack observes that the intergenerational self "grounds an individual" and "provides a larger context for understanding and dealing with life's experience(s) and challenges." Moore et al. note that such intergenerational narratives are often shaped by family historians based on stories they uncover through their research about the "struggles and successes of their ancestors" (p. 30). Such narratives serve then to help the researcher find their place in the "grand scheme of things" and become "part of the great narrative of history" (p. 30), thus working in much the same way that religious narratives do.

Moore et al. discuss how family history research can result in anchoring the sense of self more securely through connection to ancestors within a historical context, even resulting in positive attitudinal changes such as increased tolerance, empathy, and self-esteem, after researchers gain knowledge about their ancestors and greater understanding of family members. The researcher becomes "part of a long line of people who have, for example, been resilient, or creative, or struggled but overcome" (p. 24). This construction of a *narrative identity*, a life story placed into context over an even larger story, encompassing many generations, has been shown by researchers such as McAdams and McLean (2013) to have a positive effect on mental health.

Family history research can sometimes uncover "redemptive stories", where a positive outcome, such as a sense of closure, ultimately emerges from the experience of some unpleasant or distressing event. Moore et al. describe stories of this kind from their survey sample, where the family historian recounts challenges and hardships that their ancestors have overcome with fortitude and resilience, expressing astonishment and thankfulness for their persistence in the face of such challenges. They point out that learning such stories about our ancestors can serve as a reminder that "we, like them, can overcome hardship and prevail", promoting a sense of gratitude for our mere existence as a result of their tenacity, but also for the likelihood that those traits which enabled their survival "may well have been passed to us, either genetically or through family influences" (p. 55).

This relationship between participation in family research and an increased sense of gratitude might be compared to a similar correlation observed among people with religious belief, as discussed by Krause (2009) in his study demonstrating that increased church attendance and stronger God-mediated control beliefs are associated with positive changes in gratitude over time. Emmons et al. (2008) note that gratitude is an attribute that is highly valued across the world's major religions and that believers are encouraged to develop the quality. They describe it as a "recurrent religious sentiment, often reflected in gift giving and other social exchange between humans and their gods", and comment that some of the most profound gratitude experiences can be "religiously based or associated with reverent wonder and an acknowledgment of the universe, including the perception that life itself is a gift" (p. 646).

This sense of *reverence* that comes from connecting ourselves to the "whole of time", as Heintzman (2011) puts it, allows us momentarily to overcome that very human frustration with the transience of time, by recognising that "the past is still alive in the present, and the present ... is already 'pregnant' with the future" (p. 21). The storytelling tradition inherent in so many religious traditions has served, and across many communities still does serve, as a way of engendering this reverence, of bringing the past to life through the power of narrative. However, apart from these communal rituals that exist within organised religion, storytelling traditions can also evolve in a more localised setting within each family, through the individual pursuit of family history research, where perhaps it becomes its own, even more immediately relevant form of sacrament.

3. Sacred Journeys

The concept of a spiritual journey, or *pilgrimage*, is an important part of many religious traditions. The ancient site of Magadha, in north-east India, was the destination of many early practitioners of Buddhism, eager to visit the place where the Buddha was said to have lived. In Islam, faithful adherents are expected to undertake the *Hajj* at least once in their lifetime, a journey to the sacred city of Mecca that demonstrates their submission to God and solidarity with other Muslims. For Jewish people, one of the dominant stories in their sacred writings is that of the Exodus, the forty year long quest of the Israelites as they emerged from slavery in Egypt and wandered through the wilderness, searching for their promised land. Much of Jewish tradition and liturgical practice is centred around expressing this "yearning for Zion" (Langer 2018). Heintzman (2011) describes the spiritual journey at the heart of this tradition as a *mutual* quest—"the quest of God for his wayward people, and the quest of the people of Israel for their God" (p. 76).

In the Christian tradition, too, pilgrimages to Jerusalem, Rome, and other holy sites connected with the apostles, saints, and Christian martyrs, have been an important part of the religious landscape from as far back as the fourth century. Perhaps one of the most well-known Christian pilgrimages is the *Camino de Santiago* ("Way of St. James"), a set of pathways that lead to the Santiago de Compostela cathedral in Galicia, Spain, where the shrine of St. James the apostle is located, and his remains supposedly buried. Each year, hundreds of thousands of people set out to make the pilgrimage to this Cathedral, by foot, bicycle, or even on horseback (Buen Camino n.d.). Many of the travellers are of Christian background, and consider the location to be of particular religious significance. However, others simply consider the expedition to be a more generally applicable type of spiritual journey, an experience through which they can retreat from modern life and achieve inner growth.

Bowman and Sepp (2019) describe the Camino as the "prototypical" pilgrimage, particularly popular among pilgrimage first-timers. They coin the term *Caminoisation* to describe a growing set of beliefs and assumptions about pilgrimage, common among contemporary Camino pilgrims, that are increasingly becoming "transplanted and translated to other pilgrimage sites, routes and contexts" (p. 75), for instance, the idea that "the journey is more important than the destination", with pilgrimages that are undertaken on foot being considered more authentic in some sense. Bowman and Sepp comment that, in Europe particularly, the pilgrimage is seeing a revival, accompanied by a "spiritualisation of heritage" and "heritagisation of religion"—an amalgamation of the literal, physical pilgrimage with a more metaphorical kind: an internal, spiritual quest of sorts. They quote a pilgrimage service provider's observation of the modern pilgrim (p. 84):

> ... while many people no longer take part in organised religion they still recognise a spiritual dimension to their lives. They don't want the commitment or the formality of going to church but are happy to pop into a cathedral or say a quick prayer. A pilgrimage is the perfect opportunity for this sort of informal spirituality.

Heintzman also examines the idea of pilgrimage applying both internally as well as externally, noting that the entire life of religious practice can itself be construed as a journey "in search of something . . . that is never completely found", but in which the search itself can nonetheless "give direction and shape to a life" (p. 74). The *narrative* of the pilgrimage, he writes, is about learning to live life as a "journey of faith"—continuing to persevere in hope through "valleys of sorrow and loss, of doubt and despair, to the other side" (p. 83). The quest for information undertaken by family historians aligns with this notion of an internal, metaphorical pilgrimage, including the sense of it never being quite complete. Bottero (2015) notes that framing research activities as a "personal journey of self-discovery" (p. 540) is a common theme among family historians.

The "external" pilgrimage has become popular for family historians through the growing field of genealogical tourism. Shaw (2020) notes how, with "increasing globalisation, transnational migration, greater social class mobility, and what can be viewed as a depersonalized modern society, many people are exposed to a sense of social dislocation and seek to discover where 'they belong'". A literal, physical journey to uncover one's "point of origin" is one way in which this search for rootedness can take place.

Such journeys might combine historical sight-seeing with visits to more personally significant sites. Sanchini (2010) notices this diversity in the pilgrimages described by her interviewees, who "would visit the Fountain of Trevi one day and the family plot in the village cemetery the next" (p. 237). Nash (2002), too, in her work on genealogical tourists in Ireland, describes the wide variety of motives cited by her interviewees: some looking for citizenship or tax breaks, some looking to "satisfy intense longings", others with a more easy-going spirit of inquiry. She probes how questions of identity and belonging are bound up with genealogy, noting that most visitors seemed propelled by a desire to know more about "who they are" and to explore their Irishness, often hoping this desire will be satisfied through some physical experience of connection to the land (pp. 36–37).

Basu (2005, 2007), in his studies of the Scottish heritage community, found that for many people of Scottish ancestry living in other countries, visiting Scotland as a tourist allowed them to gain a sense of connection to their ancestors, thereby strengthening their own sense of self in the process. In many cases, the place they were visiting may not have been visited for generations, and yet, the for the tourist, there is still a sense of 'returning home', in which the visit "offers the dislocated self an opportunity to relocate itself both spatially and temporally" (Basu 2007, p. 9).

Moore et al. note that among their interview sample of family historians, a common theme came through of wanting to literally "walk in their ancestors' footsteps" (p. 27), seeing the things they had seen and experiencing what they had experienced. Again, we see the parallels between pilgrimages motivated by ancestry research and those journeys which might be motivated in some way by a religious belief—bringing back to mind Bowman and Sepp's notion of the "spiritualisation of heritage", as well as discussion from Taylor (2012) on pilgrimage's "malleability" (pp. 209–10):

> The plasticity and relative malleability of pilgrimage, the space it often leaves for individual and collective agency, and its ambiguous character as religious or secular activity all contribute to making it a uniquely potent way of maintaining or asserting a moral geography that reconfigures the world for personal and collective purposes.

Smith (2006) also notes this malleability of pilgrimage sites, writing that while "places, sites, objects and localities may exist as identifiable sites of heritage ... these places are not inherently valuable, nor do they carry a freight of innate meaning. Stonehenge, for instance, is basically a collection of rocks in a field" (p. 13). The value and meaning in such heritage sites, she argues, is instead bestowed by the surrounding culture and by those who visit the sites, the "activities that are undertaken at and around them, and of which they become a part" (p. 14). Through becoming connected with a culturally and socially significant event or practice, these sites symbolically take on a spiritual significance. So too for a person visiting the town their ancestors lived in, walking the streets they walked on, visiting the graveyard they are buried in—while the sites themselves may be historically unremarkable, they carry meaning and sacredness for the visiting descendant.

4. Sacred Gatherings

Sacred gatherings, involving singing, dancing, chants, and other kinds of rituals and ceremonies, have always been a part of religious practice. In ancient cultures, such rituals might be used to ward off evil spirits or appease the gods. Heintzman notes that in more modern times, while religious gatherings might retain some of the original elements of "mystery, awe, and fear", they are also more inclined to involve "elements of celebration, joy, understanding, thankfulness, and identification with the external world" (p. 25).

Adherents to religion today regularly take part in gatherings and ceremonies, usually meeting together on a weekly basis at a church, synagogue, or mosque, to connect with their community and to take part in traditional rituals that have been passed down through generations. Such rituals are known as *liturgy*—literally, "the work of the people"—an embodied participation in the sacred through collective activities such as singing, recitation of prayers and holy writings, "call and response" style readings, chanting, performing certain physical actions (such as crossing oneself in the Catholic church, or the iteration of repeated bowing in supplication in the Islamic *raka'ah* ritual), or even observing a period of silence (such as in Quaker meetings).

However, the practice of observing these types of religious ritual is waning in our modern culture. Roof notes the changing norms of society even towards the end of the last century (p. 57):

> ... many people never exposed to a religious culture, or who dropped out of churches and synagogues when they were quite young, report that when they go to religious services they often feel awkward, not sure of what to say or how to act ... [This is] less a protest of religion in the deepest sense of its meaning than a response to institutional and cultural styles that are unfamiliar or seemingly at odds with life experiences as these people know them.

While the ritual of weekly church attendance may be less common than it once was, certain kinds of liturgical practice nonetheless persist in our society. The tradition of gathering together to remember an event or mark a particular occasion is something that remains embedded in our culture. Many who no longer observe a particular religion still search for a way to regularly integrate this kind of ritualistic gathering into their lives, but without the prerequisite of belief in any god. Some research on secular Jews, for example, has demonstrated that families often still gather for Passover and Hanukah (Creese 2019; Reingold 2021). Frame (2009) comments on the tendency for secular societies to borrow religious customs in situations where they might give comfort. He discusses the example of Anzac Day commemoration services in Australia, describing them as "civic liturgies" that hold "very broad notions of the divine identity and human destiny", nonetheless leaving participants with "a reassuring sense that they have engaged in a virtuous event and rendered some spiritual service to those they commemorated" (p. 304). Taylor (2007), too, notes that people continue to be drawn to such ritualistic ceremonies both when disaster strikes and "when people feel a desire to be connected to their past". He gives the example of the mourning and funeral for Princess Diana in 1997 as an event which combined both of these motivations.

While Frame is concerned that such broadly accessible approaches to liturgy "unintentionally belittle conventional religion" and serve simply as a "veneer used to bring a little transcendence to what would otherwise appear morbid" (p. 305), the appeal of these secular/humanist liturgies seems to remain, even as participation and involvement in more formal religious rites and practices declines. Perhaps it is the sense of community and connection they bring with them, or perhaps it is the sense of awe, of observance and acknowledgement of something higher than oneself that comes with adhering to a ritual of some kind, of following a tradition observed by countless others across generations.

The family unit is perhaps one of the most natural communities among which to recreate and evolve these sacred rituals. Families most often come together to mark a celebration of some kind, for example, birthdays, weddings, graduations, and Thanksgiving. Heintzman notes that families are likely to have a favourite set of rituals and ceremonies with which to mark their shared celebration (p. 17):

> ... lighting and blowing out birthday candles, giving Uncle David the wishbone, parading from the kitchen to the living room ... [singing] "Happy Birthday," "For He's A Jolly Good Fellow," carols, campfire songs.

Such practices become their own "work of the people", their own form of liturgy. However, Heintzman also points out that not all family rituals take the form of celebration (p. 18):

> For it's in the family, above all, that we experience the most profound mysteries of life, those [that] rational thought is often helpless to explain, much less for which to offer us any real comfort: the mysteries of life and death–especially death. At funerals, wakes, and

during shivas, we summon all the resources of custom, ceremony, and ritualized family behaviour to help us bear the burden of the greatest and most painful mystery of all.

The process of learning more about our heritage through family history research can strengthen the connection we feel to family members, both past *and* present. It can increase the sense of meaning and fulfillment found by taking part in family gatherings, whether they be celebratory or mourning events. Both Kramer (2011) and Shaw (2020) discuss how family history research can provide a way to work through grief from the death of a family member, "rearranging and regenerating the meaning of the past" (Kramer 2011, p. 382), and allowing the researcher to forge and maintain a connection with those who have died.

Moore et al. discuss how sharing family history stories contributes to this strengthening of family relationships, referring to a quote found on a family reunion flyer which exemplifies the concept well (p. 52):

Have you ever wondered why we hold family reunions? The theme for our next reunion is 'Let's Stay Connected'. That is the major reason we hold reunions. Our family has grown so much and we need to get together regularly to show our mutual connection and support.

As well as connecting more strongly with family members, family historians often find their own communities in the course of their research–whether previously unknown distant family members or simply others who share an interest in genealogy. Moore et al. comment on how an interest in family history can often result in new connections to "other passionate historians", with many of their study participants having reported the friendships they had made through this shared interest, and how this had contributed to a "more positive sense of self" (p. 28). One example of such a community is the popular annual conference RootsTech, a family history convention hosted by the non-profit organisation FamilySearch. Held as an online event in 2021 due to the COVID-19 pandemic, this year the conference attracted over a million participants from all over the world, eager to connect over their shared passion (Toone 2021).

Hackstaff (2010) describes how taking part in such gatherings where stories and histories are shared can help to create new social and collective memories, allowing for the diverse representation of voices that exists among genealogists to provide "a fuller accounting of experiences that can guide our future" (p. 667). Whether it be through strengthening the existing bonds of kin, finding previously unknown family members via online searching, or forming a new kind of "family" in the form of those who share a research interest, ancestry research brings many opportunities to gather meaningfully with community.

5. Conclusions

Although in many parts of the world, over the last few decades, we have seen a clear disenchantment and disidentification with organised religion taking place, Roof (1999) comments that this is just one side of the coin. The other, in his view, is "the turning inward in search of meaning and strength" that is occurring outside the context of formal religious structures. Roof argues that many of those who have left the traditional faith of their childhood are nonetheless searching inwardly for a new sense of the sacred, "in hopes of finding a God not bound by older canons of literalism, moralism, and patriarchy, in hopes that their own biographies might yield personal insight" (p. 57). In some cases, it might be that these questioning folk look a little further afield to gain such insight, broadening their search to explore the biographies not just of themselves, but of their ancestors.

To connect with family is, as Heintzman puts it, to connect with "something larger than our individual selves, something to which we belong, and to which we have obligations, even though it's not the result of our own free choice . . . one English word that covers most of this territory is 'reverence'" (p. 18). This is all the more true for the family history researcher, whose awareness of "family" widens to include far more than their immediate kin, extending outwards both spatially and temporally to gain an understanding of different eras and different cultures from their own. A kind of reverence is experienced as a result, as new connections are found and formed between the 'other' and the self. Because this reverence comes from a sense of connectedness that is "built into all human experience", Heintzman says, "it cannot, by its *own* dynamic, stop at the boundaries of the family ... but spreads outward to the surrounding tribe, community, culture, nation, and eventually to humanity as a whole" (p. 24).

Whether through the telling and retelling of ancient stories, embarking on historical quests, or taking part in rituals and ceremonies with our kin and with like-minded people, the embodied practices that have become a part of the life of the everyday ancestry researcher are creating new understandings of the sacred, new contexts for encountering spiritual experiences, and new ways of making meaning, even through a secular lens.

Funding: This research received no external funding.

Conflicts of Interest: The author declares no conflict of interest.

Notes

[1] The moniker partially comes from the box labelled "None" on censuses and surveys that ask about religious belief. It refers in part to those who are consistently nonreligious, but also captures those people who once identified as religious but no longer do, i.e., those who are "done with church".

[2] It is worth noting that these numbers may well represent an under-reporting of non-religious people in Australia. Those who do mark a religious box on the census do not always do so because they currently believe or practise that religion, but may instead respond based on the religion of their family upbringing (Nicholls 2021). In recent years, a number of secular organisations in Australia have campaigned to encourage people who do not currently consider themselves religious to tick "no religion" on their census (see censusnoreligion.org.au, accessed on 18 August 2021), in a bid to see the census data more accurately reflect the beliefs of Australians.

[3] See Exodus 3:6, for example.

[4] Hebrews 12:1.

References

Ashton, Paul, and Paula Hamilton. 2007. *History at the Crossroads*. Ultimo: Halstead Press.
Basu, Paul. 2005. Macpherson country: Genealogical identities, spatial histories and the Scottish diasporic clanscape. *Cultural Geographies* 12: 123–50. [CrossRef]
Basu, Paul. 2007. *Highland Homecomings: Genealogy and Heritage-Tourism in the Scottish Diaspora*. London: Routledge.
Bottero, Wendy. 2015. Practising family history: 'Identity' as a category of social practice. *British Journal of Sociology* 66: 534–56. [CrossRef]
Bouma, Gary. 2006. *Australian Soul: Religion and Spirituality in the 21st Century*. Cambridge: CUP.
Bowman, Marion, and Tiina Sepp. 2019. Caminoisation and cathedrals: Replication, the heritagisation of religion, and the spiritualisation of heritage. *Religion* 49: 74–98. [CrossRef]
Buen Camino. n.d. Estadística de peregrinos del Camino de Santiago a 2018. Camino de Santiago. Available online: https://www.editorialbuencamino.com/estadistica-peregrinos-del-camino-de-santiago/ (accessed on 18 August 2021).
Carey, Hilary. 1996. *Believing in Australia: A Cultural History of Religions*. St Leonards: Allen & Unwin.
Creese, Jennifer. 2019. Secular Jewish identity and public religious participation within Australian secular multiculturalism. *Religions* 10: 69. [CrossRef]
Dissanayake, Ellen. 1988. *What Is Art for?* Seattle: University of Washington Press.
Driessnack, Martha. 2017. "Who are you from?" The importance of family stories. *Journal of Family Nursing* 23: 434–49. [CrossRef] [PubMed]
Emmons, Robert, Justin Barrett, and Sarah Schnitker. 2008. Personality and the capacity for religious and spiritual experience. In *Handbook of Personality: Theory and Research*. Edited by Oliver John, Richard Robins and Lawrence Pervin. New York: The Guilford Press, pp. 634–53.
Encyclopedia Britannica, ed. 2014. Griot. In *Encyclopedia Britannica*. Available online: https://www.britannica.com/art/griot (accessed on 18 August 2021).
Feiler, Bruce. 2013. The Stories That Bind Us. *New York Times*. March 15. Available online: http://www.nytimes.com/2013/03/17/fashion/the-family-stories-that-bind-us-this-life.html (accessed on 18 August 2021).
Frame, Tom. 2009. *Losing My Religion: Unbelief in Australia*. Sydney: University of NSW Press.
Hackstaff, Karla. 2010. Family genealogy: A sociological imagination reveals intersectional relations. *Sociology Compass* 4: 658–72. [CrossRef]
Heintzman, Ralph. 2011. *Rediscovering Reverence: The Meaning of Faith in a Secular World*. Montreal: McGill-Queen's Press.
Jacobson, Cardell. 1986. Social dislocations and the search for genealogical roots. *Human Relations* 39: 347–58. [CrossRef]

Jenkins, Kathleen. 2016. Family. In *Handbook of Religion and Society*. Edited by David Yamane. New York: Springer, pp. 219–39.
Kramer, Anne-Marie. 2011. Kinship, affinity and connectedness: Exploring the role of genealogy in personal lives. *Sociology* 45: 379–95. [CrossRef]
Krause, Neal. 2009. Religious involvement, gratitude, and change in depressive symptoms over time. *International Journal for the Psychology of Religion* 19: 155–72. [CrossRef] [PubMed]
Lambert, Ronald. 2002. Reclaiming the ancestral past: Narrative, rhetoric and the 'convict stain'. *Journal of Sociology* 38: 111–27. [CrossRef]
Langer, Ruth. 2018. Yearning for Zion in Jewish tradition. In *The Medieval Roots of Antisemitism*. Edited by Jonathan Adams and Cordelia Heß. London: Routledge, pp. 377–91.
McAdams, Dan, and Kate McLean. 2013. Narrative identity. *Current Directions in Psychological Science* 22: 233–38. [CrossRef]
Moore, Susan, Doreen Rosenthal, and Rebecca Robinson. 2021. *The Psychology of Family History: Exploring Our Genealogy*. London: Routledge.
Nash, Catherine. 2002. Genealogical identities. *Environment and Planning D: Society and Space* 20: 27–52. [CrossRef]
Nicholls, Heidi. 2021. Census time to mark 'No Religion'. *Sydney Morning Herald*. July 15. Available online: https://www.smh.com.au/national/census-time-to-mark-no-religion-20210715-p58a0w.html (accessed on 18 August 2021).
Pew Research Center. 2019. In U.S., Decline of Christianity Continues at Rapid Pace. Available online: https://www.pewforum.org/2019/10/17/in-u-s-decline-of-christianity-continues-at-rapid-pace/ (accessed on 18 August 2021).
Reingold, Matt. 2021. Secular Jewish identity in Asaf Hanuka's "The Realist". *Israel Studies* 26: 82–107. [CrossRef]
Roof, Wade Clark. 1999. *Spiritual Marketplace: Baby Boomers and the Remaking of American Religion*. Princeton: Princeton University Press.
Sanchini, Laura. 2010. Visiting La Madre Patria: Heritage pilgrimage among Montreal Italians. *Ethnologies* 32: 235–53. [CrossRef]
Shaw, Emma. 2020. "Who we are, and why we do it": A demographic overview and the cited motivations of Australia's family historians. *Journal of Family History* 45: 109–24. [CrossRef]
Smith, Laurajane. 2006. *Uses of Heritage*. London: Routledge.
Taylor, Charles. 2007. *A Secular Age*. Cambridge: Harvard University Press.
Taylor, Lawrence. 2012. Epilogue: Pilgrimage, moral geography and contemporary religion in the West. In *Gender, Nation and Religion in European Pilgrimage*. Edited by Catrien Notermans and Willy Jansen. Farnham: Ashgate, pp. 209–20.
Toone, Trent. 2021. How RootsTech Connect went from 130,000 to 1.1 million. *Deseret News*. March 3. Available online: https://www.deseret.com/faith/2021/3/3/22307976/what-drew-more-than-1-1-million-to-attend-rootstech-connect-2021-family-history-genealogy (accessed on 18 August 2021).

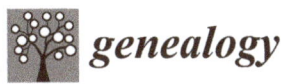

genealogy

Article

(Re)discovering the Familial Past and Its Impact on Historical Consciousness

Emma L. Shaw * and Debra J. Donnelly

School of Education, College of Human & Social Futures, The University of Newcastle, Callaghan, NSW 2308, Australia; Debra.donnelly@newcastle.edu.au
* Correspondence: emma.shaw@newcastle.edu.au

Abstract: Family history has become a significant contributor to public and social histories exploring and (re)discovering the micro narratives of the past. Due to the growing democratisation of digital access to documents and the proliferation of family history media platforms, family history is now challenging traditional custodianship of the past. Family history research has moved beyond the realms of archives, libraries and community-based history societies to occupy an important space in the public domain. This paper reports on some of the findings of a recent study into the historical thinking and research practices of Australian family historians. Using a case study methodology, it examines the proposition that researching family history has major impacts on historical understanding and consciousness using the analytic frameworks of Jorn Rüsen's Disciplinary Matrix and his Typology of Historical Consciousness. This research not only proposes these major impacts but argues that some family historians are shifting the historical landscape through the dissemination of their research for public consumption beyond traditional family history audiences.

Keywords: historical consciousness; family history research; family historians; temporal orientation; case study

Citation: Shaw, Emma L., and Debra J. Donnelly. 2021. (Re)discovering the Familial Past and Its Impact on Historical Consciousness. *Genealogy* 5: 102. https://doi.org/10.3390/genealogy5040102

Received: 25 October 2021
Accepted: 25 November 2021
Published: 1 December 2021

Publisher's Note: MDPI stays neutral with regard to jurisdictional claims in published maps and institutional affiliations.

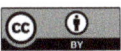

Copyright: © 2021 by the authors. Licensee MDPI, Basel, Switzerland. This article is an open access article distributed under the terms and conditions of the Creative Commons Attribution (CC BY) license (https://creativecommons.org/licenses/by/4.0/).

1. Introduction

Family history research is rapidly changing, and influencing, the historical landscape. This multi-billion-dollar industry sees millions of people around the world researching and (re)discovering their familial pasts. Revolutionised by technological advances, family history research has moved beyond the realms of archives, libraries and community-based history societies to occupy an important space in the public domain. Today we see family history represented across multiple media platforms intended for popular consumption such as investigative television, docudramas, advertising spaces, and DNA testing sites to name a few (Donnelly and Shaw 2020). Coupled with the proliferation of websites and databases, in addition to how-to books, magazines, and thousands of social media groups and family history societies worldwide, family history research has become a global phenomenon.

Consequentially, family histories have become an important contributor to public and social histories exploring and publicising the micro narratives of the past. Burgeoned by widely available historical information, and a growing democratisation of digital access to documents, the family history 'boom' represents an historiographic shift in the perceived custodianship of the past. Family historians, once considered to be the 'poor cousins' of academic historians, are now widely consulted by those in the academy in the (re)creation of local, social, public and other histories (Evans 2021). While family historians are often self-taught, many are able to draw on historical research methodologies, and are skilled and flexible in locating, corroborating, and contextualising a vast array of sources in the compilation of their familial narratives (Kramer 2011; Evans 2021; Shaw 2020). Such narratives shift between the familial and the broader historical sphere, as the past is reformed and retold, and thus present a diverse range of alternative historical perspectives.

This paper reports on some of the findings of a recent study into the historical thinking and research practices of Australian family historians. Using a case study methodology, we examine the proposition that some family historians are mirroring the work of academic historians and developing advanced historical consciousness by considering their disciplinary practices and understandings through an analytic alignment with Jorn Rüsen's Disciplinary Matrix (Rüsen 1993) and his Typology of Historical Consciousness (Rüsen 1996). Rüsen is a well-known as a philosopher of history and is particularly interested in the role of history in intersection between the past and present. His disciplinary matrix, examines the part played by issues of motives, functions, theories, representations, and methods, and allows for the investigation of both the ontological and practical aspects of family history research. Applying this matrix and the typology to the selected case studies is an important way to see how family history research impacts on an individual's relationship to, and understandings of, the past which is commonly referred to as an historical consciousness.

2. Conceptualising Historical Consciousness

Since the 1970s, much scholarly interest has focussed on the formation of historical consciousness and the ways that researchers construct narratives to understand themselves as historical beings, orientated in place and time (Seixas 2006). The influential German philosopher Hans-Georg Gadamer (1977) characterises historical consciousness as a cultural manifestation with a specific locality in space and time, claiming "historical consciousness no longer listens sanctimoniously to the voice that reaches out from the past but, in reflection on it, replaces it within the context where it took root in order to see the significance and relative value proper to it" (p. 9). More recently, Swedish academic Robert Thorpe (2014) explained, "at the most fundamental level a historical consciousness is manifested through narratives, and these narratives can be applied to uses of history on an individual level and historical culture on a societal or public level" (p. 19). This aligns with Rüsen's (2004) views of historical consciousness "as a synthesis of moral and temporal consciousness" (p. 78) arguing our reactions to any given situation depends on our socially constructed sense of morality, and what we know contextually and historically about a situation. Rüsen views our historical consciousness as "a necessary prerequisite" to navigate the present and to plan for the future (p. 66).

In his work on historical consciousness, Rüsen (1996, 2006) developed a typology, which identified and outlined four types of historical consciousness: *traditional*; *exemplary*; *critical*; and *genetic* historical consciousness. He argued that the principals of 'tradition' is grounded in meaning and sense-making which remain the most popular and the most frequently used and provide a "cultural orientation for practical human life using certain reference to the past" (p. 46). He further insists that tradition is "the starting point for every development of historical consciousness" (p. 50). *Exemplary* historical consciousness uses events in the past to provide general rules that can be applied to similar cases in the present. *Critical* historical consciousness is more sophisticated in that the individual understands that much truth in history is reliant on point of view, yet do not view themselves as historical beings. The final stage of the Typology Rüsen calls *Genetic* historical consciousness. Here, the individual understands how knowledge is a construction that changes over time and that historical evidence requires contextualisation. As Thorpe (2014) argues, "an individual that has no understanding of the contextual contingency of history cannot make a genetic use of history". (p. 21). Peter Seixas (2006) used Rüsen's Typology as a heuristic to further explore the discipline of history. A synopsis is presented in Table 1 below.

Table 1. Epistemic qualities of historical consciousness (adapted from Seixas 2006, pp. 145–49).

Types of Historical Consciousness	Understanding History
Traditional	• Epistemologically rudimentary • No means for a critical assessment of history or historical accounts • No means for treating contradictory accounts of history
Exemplary	• Turns history into a positivist science • Values (such as 'human rights') are historically derivative • Treats historical account as substantive, yet engages with how to verify or falsify historical claims
Critical	• Questions the possibility of truth in history • Does not offer a method of how to treat history, apart from falsifying or verifying its accounts • Displays an inability to historicise the point of the researcher
Genetic	• Displays an appreciation that knowledge is constructed by a community of inquiry • Historical knowledge changes over time and must be contextually bound to the historical era in which it was created • False and true historical accounts are treated with complexity

Therefore, historical consciousness is more than how we think about the past. It is linked to personal and cultural identity and is influenced by "all things historical" (Rüsen 2004, p. viii). An individual's historical consciousness is potentially influenced and enhanced by engaging in historical research activities such as investigating one's family history or undertaking study of history in a formal institution of learning, both of which involve the creation of historical outputs, such as essays, books, and family trees. These historical understandings often spill into interests and pastimes, such as reading historical novels, watching with historical films and documentaries, attending museums, watching historically themed television programmes, travelling to places of historical significance. Rüsen's Disciplinary Matrix links disciplinary knowledge and history in everyday life, while his typology serves to describe various types of historical consciousness. Lee (2004) makes the important point that the Typology is not a "ladder-like progression" (p. 5) with each stage building on the former, but that the stages can co-exist and change depending on the individuals' encounter with the past.

3. Research Design and Case Study as a Methodology

This research reports on part of the findings of a larger qualitiative study investigating the research practices and historical thinking and consciousness of Australian family historians (Shaw 2020). Qualitative research involves collecting an analysing non-numerical data through an analysis of investigative methods such as interviews, observations, and open-response survey questions (Creswell 2012). It focuses on gaining insight an understanding of an individual's perceptions and understandings of their lived experience. The study used a tri-phase design comprised of survey (n = 1406), semi-structured interviews (n = 11) and the development of four in-depth case studies. The triangulated case study data were aligned to Rüsen's Disciplinary Matrix and the case studies' historical consciousness were framed against the Typology of Historical Consciousness to explore their practical and theoretical workings as historians, which form the focus of this paper.

Qualitative case study design is appropriate for this paper as it allows the researchers to draw from the wisdom and insight of those who have experienced family history research and understand its impact on perceptions of the present. "One selects a case study approach because one wishes to understand the particular in depth" (Merriam 1998, p. 173). Case studies are examples of purposeful sampling and present an in-depth study of exemplary "information-rich cases" (Sandelowski 1995, p. 180). Case study, as a research methodology, is commonly defined as "an in-depth exploration of a bounded system (activity, event, process, or individuals) based on extensive data collection" (Creswell 2012, p. 465; Stake 1995). A bounded system means that the case is separated out for research in terms of time, place or some physical boundaries (Creswell 2012). The case studies in this project were bounded in time being examples of family historians in the early 21st century and by location all living and working in Australia. They are all examples of single case designs which are used to confirm or challenge a theory, or to represent a unique or extreme case (Yin 1989).

Yin (1989) defines case study is "an empirical inquiry ... when the boundaries between phenomenon and context are not clearly evident; and in which multiple sources of evidence are used" (p. 23). Single-case designs require careful investigation to avoid misrepresentation and to maximise the investigator's access to the evidence. Each individual case study consists of a "whole" study, in which facts are gathered from various sources and conclusions drawn on those facts (Tellis 1997), and are not selected for the purposes of generalisability (Lincoln and Guba 2000; Stake 1995). "It [a case study] provides a slice from the lifeworld that is the proper subject matter for the interpretivist inquirer ... every topic must be seen as carrying its own logic, sense and order, structure and meaning" (Denzin 2005, pp. 133–34).

These case studies exemplify distinctive approaches to family history investigation. The voices of the family history researchers are a vital element in these case studies, and direct quotations from the data are a feature of the reported findings. The voices of the participants in the cases are added to that of the researchers, so providing the reader with a more vivid and nuanced account (Tellis 1997). By adopting this approach, the researchers were able to share the practitioner experience and learn about their family history investigative practices and its impact on their sense of the past and the impact of this on their lives.

The case study subjects were volunteers selected from the interviewees. Their survey and interview responses were used as a means of identifying accomplished researchers, with diverse interests and outputs. All indicated a strong interest in history more broadly, but the motives for commencing their familial research varied markedly. The case study subjects reflected the gender imbalance and ethnic homogeneity of the survey respondents. Three case study subjects identified as female, and one identified as a male. All identified as Anglo-Celtic, but were diverse in that they represented different demographics in age, location, research experience, and hours dedicated to familial research. They had studied at the tertiary level, and except Jane, had studied disciplinary history at high school. Jane was formally trained in historical research methodologies, and the others were self-taught family history researchers. All the case study subjects shared their discoveries with family and John, Jane, and Claire were published authors. A synopsis of the case study subjects is presented in Table 2 below.

Table 2. Demographic overview of case study participants.

	Gender	Age	Highest Level of Education	Profession	Level of History Studies	Year FH Was Started	Hours per Week	Membership of Historical Society	Publication of Findings
John	male	46	Bachelor degree	HR consultant	- school	1980s + 2013	1–40+	yes	yes
Jane	female	41	Postgraduate coursework	Educational administrator	- school - university	2000	20	yes	yes
Lucy	female	25	Postgraduate coursework	Lawyer	- school	2005	5	no	no
Claire	female	69	Postgraduate coursework	Science teacher	- school	1984	20+	yes	yes

4. Rüsen's Disciplinary Matrix as an Analytical Tool

Rüsen (1993) developed a Disciplinary Matrix which embraces five central factors or principles of historical thinking: the cognitive interest of human beings in having an orientation in time; theories or "leading views" concerning the experiences of the past; empirical research methods; forms of representation; and the function of offering orientation to society (Megill 1994). Within the matrix, Theories (*conceptions of history*), Methods (*the tools used for empirical work*), and Forms of representation (*what does the result of the historical inquiry look like*) are illustrative of engagement with the history discipline. Interests (*societal need for temporal orientation*) and Functions (*what does the historical inquiry do with regard to identity construction and temporal guidance*) relate to 'life practice'.

Rüsen's Disciplinary Matrix (Rüsen 1993) describes the relationship between disciplinary historical knowledge and history in contemporary life, and how these contribute to the development of historical consciousness. The Disciplinary Matrix offers a flexible model in which to analyse how individuals interact with the discipline of history and their motivations for doing so. As Gosselin (2012) contends, "the strength of Rüsen's model lies in its ability to recognise the relationship between the internal logic of the historical discipline and everyday life" (p. 59). Chapman (2014) concludes that Rusen's matrix can be useful diagnostically as a tool for identifying dimensions of historical interpretation and he suggests "pedagogies informed by kind of thinking embodied in the matrix can be helpful for progressing historical thinking" and that "Rüsen's model is a valuable tool for organising reflection on historiography and on accounts of historical practice." (p. 70). The matrix is represented diagrammatically in Figure 1 below.

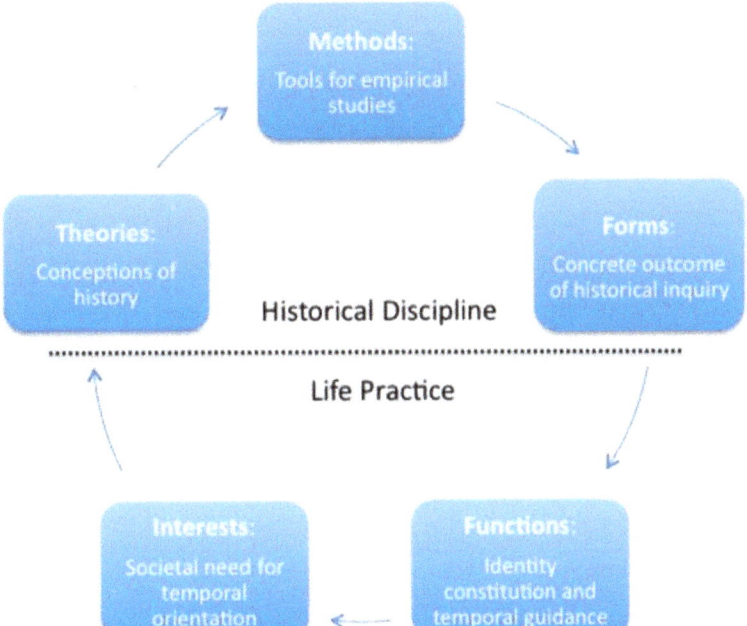

Figure 1. Jorn Rüsen's Disciplinary Matrix (Rüsen 1993).

The case studies in this paper were examined in alignment with the central factors of the matrix, and questions were developed to guide the analytic process as outlined in Table 3 below. Rüsen's matrix has been modified and individualised for each of the four case studies to determine the impact of family history research and its relationship to historical consciousness. These adapted diagrammatical representations, presented as Figures 2–5, facilitate comparing and contrasting of the case studies.

Table 3. Guiding analytic questions in alignment with the Disciplinary Matrix.

Rüsen's Disciplinary Matrix	Guiding Analytic Questions
1. Interest in orientation in time.	What is the family history researchers interested in (re)discovering? What are the motivations?
2. Theories or conceptions of history:	How does the family history researcher define history? What does it mean to interpret the past?
3. Tools and methodologies used for empirical work	How does the family history researcher explore emergent questions and themes about the past?
4. Forms of historical representation	In what ways does the family history researcher convey their historical argument and/or discoveries. What are the main ideas coming from the research?
5. Function of identity construction and temporal guidance.	What impacts do these new discoveries and understandings of the familial past have in terms of identity formation and temporal guidance?

- Case study 1: John (pseudonym), 46 Year-old HR consultant.

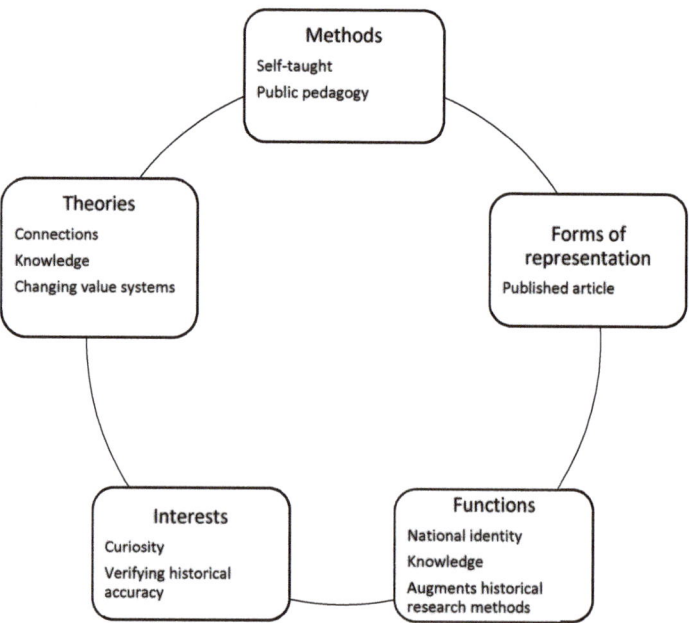

Figure 2. Case study one in alignment with Rüsen's (1993) Disciplinary Matrix.

John lives in New South Wales, Australia. His highest level of educational attainment is a bachelor's degree, and he had only formally studied history at school. He currently spends up to 40 h per week researching his family history and is a member of a historical society. John commenced his family history research in 1979 citing "simple **interest**" but explained that "you didn't know what was available ... it was like staring into a big black hole, not knowing what to look for or what was available, or how to go about it". He recommenced his research in 2013 when he uncovered a family connection to a famous

Australian artwork, and through his research, was able to challenge the written history of a painting of national significance. He tells that

Back when I first started in 1979, I initially spoke to my mother [about the painting]. In addition, it was only 30 years later, when I started to discover and piece together the big puzzle, and I found that . . . everything she said, it all fitted in.

John also revealed an **interest** in acquiring an increase in familial knowledge as he reported "I needed to understand not just how, not just the story of [name] in it, and what came before him, and also what came after him, to understand what happened with the land. And I also wanted to know how he acquired land". This meant investigating and eventually correcting an established historical narrative. He spoke of contextualising his research, and explained "It was only by doing that research of not just this narrow, looking down onto [name] but what was around him" that led to a deeper understanding of the past.

John's **theory of history** was an intense personalisation of the past. Of the painting he said "What I see is my great-uncle. What I see are his cows, and what I see in the background behind him is the shadow of the peppercorn trees the homestead where my great-grandfather was born. And when you start thinking about that, it's, wow. And they lived in this house". Here John illuminates a strong affective connection to this historical artefact. Unlike the other case studies subjects the main thrust of his research is centred on the people around the painting, as opposed to a structured and complete family tree.

John is a self-taught historical researcher but deftly draws upon various **methods** to develop his family history. In an act of public pedagogy, where learning is seen as "the informal learning and ever educational experiences occurring within popular culture, popular media, and everyday life" (Freishtat and Sandlin 2010, p. 503) he learned to research in and across multiple digital media platforms in addition to informal sites of education such as libraries, archives, museums, and art galleries. John confessed that he felt quite lost when commencing his genealogical journey and increased his skills by trial and error as time progressed. John spoke of using "many, many different guides" and countless websites. He referred to his local library which "has an excellent reference section" and speaking to historians at the archives.

John demonstrated flexibility in his research **methods.** He "let the painting tell the story" and started by comparing the geographical features of paintings by the same artist and then "looked at parish maps" which led to the use of conveyancing documents and a will. He was able to find out that his ancestor lived in "a two room hut" by exploring probate documents for their estates, which was supported by a "description in the coroner's inquest". Despite being self-taught in historical research, John showed agility in his application of a variety of research apparatuses. He used multiple sources of evidence and recognised the importance of historical context by explaining "I think what it's taught me is that a lot of bad things happened back then. And you've got to realise that the values that we have now, aren't the values that were around at that time. And you then have to start looking at things as to how they looked at things back then".

The **form of representation** of John's research is a widely distributed article outlining the history of an important Australian painting. There has been previous works written of the painting but as John explained "where are the supporting facts? And there weren't any, it was just someone telling a story". He continued by arguing that he "could've written a document which was literally tearing apart paragraph by paragraph, but that would have just ended up being an article which was us against them . . . which wouldn't have proved anything". He has given talks about his research at the National Art Gallery of Australia, and has located and met the descendents of the artist.

John's family history research **functioned** to strengthen his connection with society, "hard to say how, but I find I can relate more to the history of the country". Another **function** of his research was that his wider historical knowledge had intensified due to his family history research. His research also **functioned** to provide him with a deeper appreciation of the present, to understand the past and his historical consciousness was augmented by his historical investigations. This aligns with critical historical consciousness of Rüsen's Typology, in that he is interested in exploring the past to verify historical accounts.

- Case study 2: Jane (pseudonym), 41 year-old education administrator

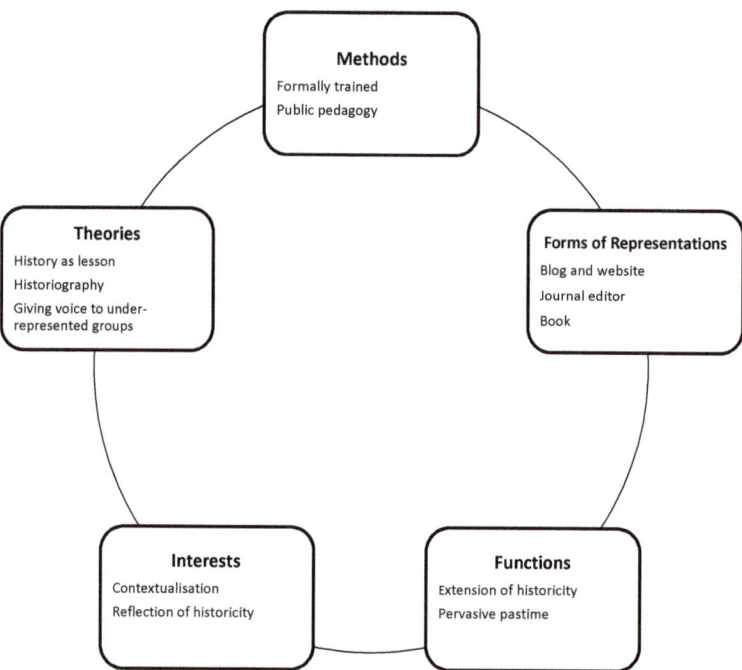

Figure 3. Case study two in alignment with Rüsen's (1993) Disciplinary Matrix.

Jane originally from Victoria, but now resides in New South Wales, Australia. She identifies as Australian with an Anglo-Celtic ethnic cultural background. She is highly educated, having completed a postgraduate coursework degree, and she cites 'education administration' as her occupation. She has been undertaking her family history research for sixteen years and dedicates an average of twenty hours per week to her research. She has studied history as an academic subject at several levels from compulsory history at school to senior history at school and senior extension history at school and then onto university studies with a major in History.

When asked about her **theories of history**, Jane explained that "It means the study of everything that has contributed to who I am and what the society I live in is and it's something I find very enjoyable to both produce and participate in". For Jane the study of history is about locating herself in time and orientating her life in society. It also meant attention to the disciplinary aspects of historical inquiry, and was a passion to be simultaneously consumed and produced. When asked about her evolving understand of history as a discipline, Jane pointed to a shift from grand in focus to micro-historical narratives within historical scholarship. She acknowledged the recent shift to view history as multi-voiced, with the inclusion of previously marginal historical voices, such as social, women's, indigenous and immigrant histories. Janes successfully locates herself firmly within the contemporary historical climate:

"I think that's just been a natural trend in historical research for the last 40 years anyway, with the rise of indigenous history and religious history and ethnic history, and whatever else, all the people, all the different groups that have been left out of the more traditional big picture, important people, dates type history ... It's not so much that the history's changed; it's the way that people look at the history that's changed."

Jane further emphasised the importance of history to contemporary understandings and used a very relevant example, although this interview was held before the COVID Pandemic. She believes that as humans we benefit from learning the lessons of history. As such, Jane saw history as having a didactic purpose and she explains one impact on her historical consciousness from her exploration of history. Jane when searching a parish register for ancestral names when she happened upon a large number of children dying of measles:

[This is an] example of how history impacts on modern life is the anti-vaxers [anti-vaccinations] people of today. Because anyone that's spent any time doing family history I think would just want to grab these people around the throat and throttle them ... my solution with these people is to drag them to a town of a 19th century cemetery, and make them sit there and read out the gravestone of every kid under the age of five who died of these diseases, and make them do it until they change their mind.

Jane's historical research **methods** are well developed. Jane is experienced in historical inquiry methodologies acquired through assorted encounters with history as an academic discipline as well as a wide range of learning opportunities focussed on family history research. She cites a wide range a university genealogy course, family history magazines, genealogical television programmes, personal practice, interaction with other family history researchers, participation in online communities, and family history how-to books.

Jane is an established family historian working in various **forms of representation**. Jane writes a newsletter about family history courses and events, is the editor of the historical society journal, maintains blog and website about family history research methods, and is involved in writing a book in collaboration with the university academics.

Following on from her school and university History studies, Jane has undertaken the role of teacher and mentor to many family and local history researchers. She runs research methodology courses and as such has taken on the role of public pedagogue. Jane is very involved in her historical society being the secretary and journal editor. She is currently working on two projects about World War One soldiers of her local area.

Jane expressed her frustration at the lack of archival organisation within the society, revealing she shouldered the responsibility of attempting to introduce orderliness to the documents and artefacts collected by the society over time.

It's the regular story of most historical societies; it's a very ageing demographic in membership. It's a small society anyway, and it's getting smaller as people basically die, and it's very hard to attract new members.

Jane's leisure activities further highlight her **interest** in history. She reported that as well as her local historical society work, she undertakes a wide-ranging interest in public history activities such as viewing historical movies and documentaries on television, reading historical non-fiction books, regularly attending museums. She is interested in her family research in its historical context and has a deep understanding of how history influences the present. She sees her family history research as confirmation of her historicity, meaning authenticity based on verifiable evidence.

Jane's historical consciousness has a strong influence on her values, who she is, and how she perceives herself. Her historical activities and practices **function** as a reflection of her historical ideologies, and she actively produces historical representations and seeks scholarship to support and augment her historical experiences in their totality. Janes' interest in history is all-pervasive as it encompasses, and permeates, all aspects of her life as she claims, "Oh if I win lotto, my life is going to be going from archive to archive ... just jumping into the documents. I could do that for weeks on end, that's not a problem." Jane's historical consciousness is nuanced and sophisticated and with an understanding that time and values systems change over time, placing her at genetic historical consciousness in Rüsen's Typology.

- Case study 3: Lucy (pseudonym), 25 year-old lawyer

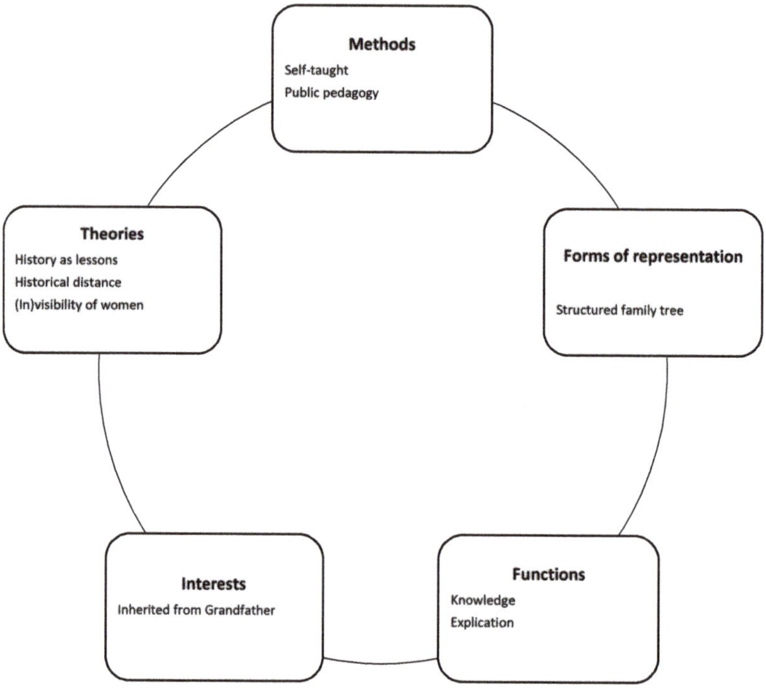

Figure 4. Case study three in alignment with Rüsen's (1993) Disciplinary Matrix.

Diagram contents:
- **Methods**: Self-taught; Public pedagogy
- **Forms of representation**: Structured family tree
- **Functions**: Knowledge Explication
- **Interests**: Inherited from Grandfather
- **Theories**: History as lessons; Historical distance; (In)visibility of women

Lucy is from Sydney, New South Wales. She is currently completing her PhD in law, and she studied history in high school. She commenced her family history research when she was 13, and she is not a member of a historical society. She has no plans to publish her family history research at this time. Lucy cited her grandfather as the catalyst for her **interest** in family history research. She explained that he "had started up his family tree and so he would tell us, my brothers and I, some family stories. And he passed on the family tree to me because he thought I might be interested and that's what sort of started it off". As time progressed, her interest became a desire "to get a fuller picture of where my family came from", which culminated in a comprehensive family tree which is the **form of representation** of her research.

Lucy is also self-taught in historical research **methods**. She told that "it was really trial and error and Googling ... because I think back when I started there wasn't really a great deal of things online that were freely available as there are now". She spoke of how her research **methods** grew over time, and of the collegiality of the online genealogical community which "helped out". She told how she cross-referencing her sources, and ensured their accuracy through a "process of elimination". Lucy further revealed that she contextualised her findings within the broader historical landscape by initially thinking about "the legal connections" and cited the Matrimonial Clauses Act (1858) and Lord Hardwicke's Act (1753), and of the **methods** she used to break through 'brick walls'.

Antithetically to other case studies in this paper, Lucy's family history research did not **function** to create an affective relationship to her family past. She claimed her research has not impacted on her life, and she explicitly told of an impassive emotional connection to her ancestral past, despite her interest. She explained that "I could say I don't get horrified when I read things. Like you know in those *Who Do You Think You Are?* programmes you find the celebrities crying over small things about what their ancestor's gone through? I don't get emotionally attached like that". She explained that temporal distance, defined as "a position of detached observation made possible by the passage of time" (Phillips 2011, p. 11) was the reason why she could not connect with her ancestors by stating "I try to take an objective view towards what I look at because there is a distance between us. I don't feel completely connected with them, but I'm interested in finding out about them".

Lucy's research, however, did **function** to provide her with knowledge of the past and connect her to an estranged part of her family. She explained that "my parents divorced when I was very young, so I didn't have much contact with my Dad's family ... and it was really trying to bridge that gap". Another **function** of her research was to provide explanation as a means of understanding the perspectives of the people of the past, and to help to make sense of and explain their actions in both the past and the present. She revealed "And he was from a very poor Irish family and he used to walk to school barefoot and so it sort of gives you an impression of why he might have become a hardened person, because of his upbringing and the way he was treated".

Lucy's **theories of history** were well-defined, and her historical consciousness is best described in Rüsen's Typology as genetic. Lucy understands the constructed nature of history and spoke of the invisibility of women in older historical accounts and argued "it does disappoint me when I can't find out anything about some of my female convicts, because they're as much of my history as the men". She **theorised** history as a pedagogical tool in which the past "helps us reflect on what we should be doing in the present or the future to see what might have worked or might not have worked in the past, and how that might have influenced now, or what we should do in the future. It's a reflective exercise and you like to see what people in the past did, or events that happened in the past and how that's shaped us". Again, this reasoning is evidence of Lucy's high-level historical consciousness, as the past is used to understanding the present and considers its impact on the future.

- Case study 4: Claire (pseudonym), 68 year-old teacher

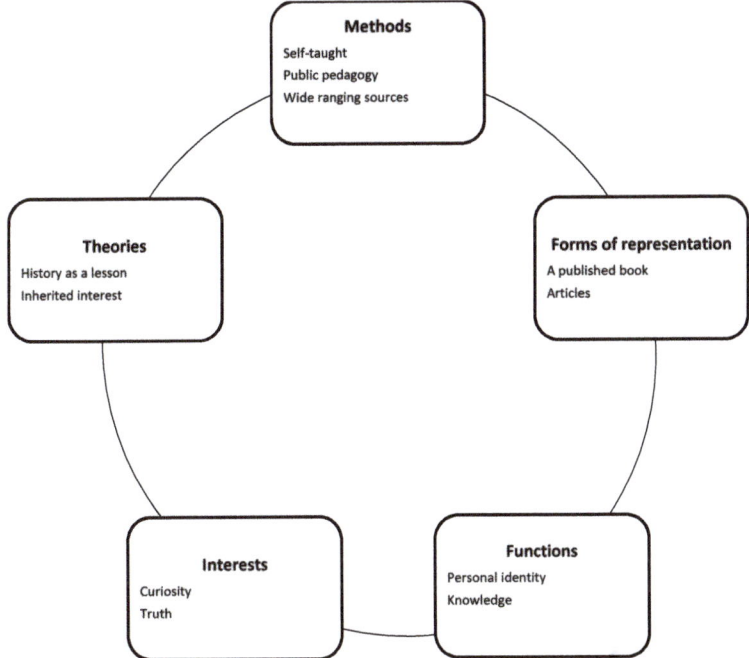

Figure 5. Case study four in alignment with Rüsen's (1993) Disciplinary Matrix.

Claire is from Queensland, Australia. She identifies as Australian, with European ethnic and/or cultural background. She is highly educated having completed a coursework Masters degree, and is a science teacher in a secondary high school where she is Head of her Department. Claire is a very experienced family history researcher having commenced her familial research in 1984 and dedicates a maximum of 20 h per week on her family history research.

Claire is **interested** in history in many forms and is prompted by curiosity and a search for "truth." She views historical movies and documentaries on television, and she reads historical non-fiction books. "I'm one of those people who doesn't read fiction, so it's either history or autobiographies, or science books or something". Claire participated at a local historical society and explained that she was motivated by her research quest. "I just go out there if I wanna do research". She had not taken on special offices or duties within the society, but expressed an interest in doing so when she retires. As to **forms of representation** of her work, Claire wrote two articles for the society that had been published in their newsletter. Her **methods** of historical research are mainly self-taught. In the beginning, her research journey was ad hoc in its approach, and when interviewed and asked how she learned to 'do' her research, she stated:

> It was a bit hard when I started ... because there was nothing online, there was no such thing as the internet. I used to go out to the Mormons, and they were very helpful, and I was using German records a lot, and they would get the film in and I'd sit there and read it painstakingly. Oh, and we used to go to the archives ... it was very, very time consuming."

Over the years Claire has developed advanced research skills in virtual and real contexts and has acquired the skills to locate, select, apply, and corroborate various and diverse historical sources.

> I try to build up a picture of the person's life and see how it fits together, and usually you can find where the discrepancy is. You've gotta look at them in context, and you've gotta look at the bigger picture ... you can't sometimes just go to what you're tryin' to find out ... if it doesn't fit in, then it's not right is it?

An interesting revelation to emerge in the interview was that Claire had travelled internationally to Germany and Scotland to conduct her family history research. The literature refers to this as genealogical tourism (Santos and Yan 2009). With regard to Scotland, Claire talked of how her ancestors were cleared from the Highlands and "they were told to become fishermen, and it's such ... we visited up there and it's such barren sort of awful country, it'd be very hard to exist". In Scotland, she visited the village from which her ancestors came, and saw the house where they lived, which was, in her words, "quite thrilling". In Germany, Claire took many of the photographs featured in her book and it was this German family that was the basis of her book—another **form of representation** which had some modest success commercially.

When asked about her **theories of history**, Claire defined history as "events that are past—usually long past". Probed further in the interview about her interest in history more generally, she replied that "I think you can learn a lot from it really". Locating her interest in history to a familial trait, she mused that "I s'pose my mother was always interested in history, I might get it from her. I just think you learn a lot from history, and it helps you understand the world around you a lot better". As an example, she divulged that she had just finished reading a book about New Guinea during the Second World War. Her reason for doing so was an attempt to understand and contextualise her father's wartime experience as he was stationed there during the war. She told of how he always hated the Japanese, and "he went to his grave hating them".

When asked about her **theories of history**, Claire acknowledged that her family history research allowed her to see the importance of contextualisation:

> I don't think you can research people without looking at the history behind it ... because it affects them so much, doesn't it? Everyday life and what they did and

why they did it ... that's probably why I got interested in history, trying to put them into context.

Claire's contextualisation of her ancestors into their wider political and social milieus served an important **function** in her understanding of herself as an historical being. She located her ancestors in place and time, and sought to comprehend the actions and motives of people of the past through exploring the social/political/economic elements of the time period being researched. This process augmented her historical understanding and has led Claire to a greater understanding of her own life, and who she is as a person. While not being formally schooled in the conceptual underpinnings of the history discipline, Claire reveals a sophisticated approach to her research and a well-developed historical consciousness which can be aligned to genetic in Rüsen's Typology.

5. Conclusions

Each of the examined case study subjects is unique in their very different contexts backgrounds, ages and professions. However, the subjects in this study were all skilled at locating, corroborating, and contextualising historical sources to compile and disseminate historical accounts. The case study subjects were historically minded individuals who devoted considerable time to their family history research activities. All were enthusiastic about their research which attests to the strong personal connection that develops between the family history researcher and their ancestors. Through a process of trial and error, they had developed agile approaches to overcoming research obstacles. They used a variety of research apparatus shifting between archival and digital platforms and had established reciprocal connections with family history communities. With the exception of Jane, all learned their family history research skills in a public setting, with little tutoring from formalised institutions of learning. While they reported different motives for commencing their family history research, Lucy, Claire, and John were inspired by their family members' interest in the past. Lucy was inspired to continue her grandfather's research while John was motivated to investigate his family connection to a well-known colonial painting to confirm his mother's familial narrative. Claire saw her interest in history as a family trait which was passed to her from her mother. Jane's interest grew from her early encounters with history at school.

Through enacting historical research processes to develop narratives, they learned of the importance of contextualisation of historical accounts, and were shown to have a sophisticated historical consciousness. As shown in Jane's concluding statement, "For me, history is important. My research has helped me see its impact on modern life". They claim that this changed the ways they thought about the past, increased their historically related activities, and enhanced their understanding of the disciplinary nuances. Jane and Lucy were aware of current trend in historiographic discourses which sees a focus on previously marginalised voices. Claire travelled widely to confirm the stories of her family past and contextualised these to produce a published book. Lucy, Jane, and Claire's understanding of contextualisation and varying perspectives, which aligns with a genetic historical consciousness. John's research was less concerned with contextualisation but allowed him to critique and rewrite an established historical account and become an acknowledged authority in his field of investigation. His historical consciousness was categorised as critical as he sought to test and challenge accepted historical narratives.

This study asserts that family histories can be important contributors to public history, and that some family history researchers can be considered historians, despite being predominantly self-taught in historical research methodologies. All the case study subjects produced historical accounts of their research findings which took forms of family trees, journal articles, and monographs. With the exception of Lucy, these works have been disseminated for public consumption and education.

These case studies illustrate that family history research can become an agent for the evolution of an historical consciousness as theorised by Rüsen's Disciplinary Matrix and evidenced by his typology. By undertaking their research quests these individuals' relationships with the past can be seen to be enhanced through investigation and discovery. The ancestors and narratives they uncovered became part of their family story, as opposed to being distant historical happenings peopled by strangers. All four case study subjects reported their family history research gave them insight into historical research and writing and changed their sense of self. Learning about their families' past, the experiences of their ancestors, and contextualising these in a broader historical setting impacted on their identities, their pastimes, and their historical understanding. This research found that the historical consciousness of all the case study subjects was substantially augmented by their family history research.

Author Contributions: Conceptualization, E.L.S.; methodology, D.J.D.; formal analysis, E.L.S. and D.J.D.; investigation, E.L.S.; writing—original draft preparation, E.L.S. and D.J.D.; writing—review and editing, D.J.D. and E.L.S.; All authors have read and agreed to the published version of the manuscript.

Funding: This research received no external funding.

Institutional Review Board Statement: This project has been approved by the University's Human Research Ethics Committee, Approval No. H-2014-0353.

Informed Consent Statement: Informed consent was obtained from all subjects involved in the study.

Data Availability Statement: Not applicable.

Conflicts of Interest: The authors declare no conflict of interest.

References

Chapman, Arthur. 2014. "But it might not just be their political views": Using Jorn Rusen's Disciplinary Matrix to develop understandings of historical interpretation. *Caderno de Pesquisa: Pensamento Educacional* 9: 67–85.
Creswell, John. 2012. *Educational Research*. Boston: Pearson.
Denzin, Norman. 2005. Emancipatory discourses and the ethics and politics of interpretation. In *Handbook of Qualitative Research*. Edited by Norman Denzin and Yvonna Lincoln. Thousand Oaks: Sage.
Donnelly, Debra, and Emma Shaw. 2020. Docudrama as histotainment: Repackaging family history in the digital age. *Public History Review* 27: 48–68. [CrossRef]
Evans, Tanya. 2021. Family history: Community and collaboration. In *Family History and Historians in Australia and New Zealand*. Edited by Malcolm Allbrook and Sophie Scott-Brown. New York: Routledge, pp. 197–207.
Freishtat, Richard, and Jennfier Sandlin. 2010. Shaping youth discourse about technology: Technological colonization, manifest destiny, and the frontier myth in Facebook's public pedagogy. *Educational Studies: A Journal of the American Educational Studies Association* 46: 503–23. [CrossRef]
Gadamer, Hans-Georg. 1977. The universality of the hermeneutical problem. In *Philosophical Hermeneutics*. Translated by David Linge. Los Angeles: University of California Press.
Gosselin, Viviane. 2012. Open to Interpretation: Mobilizing Historical Thinking in the Museum. Unpublished doctoral dissertation, University of British Columbia, Vancouver, BC, Canada.
Kramer, Anne-Marie. 2011. Kinship, affinity and connectedness: Exploring the role of genealogy in personal lives. *Sociology* 45: 379–45. [CrossRef]
Lee, Peter. 2004. 'Walking backwards into tomorrow'. Historical consciousness and understanding history. *International Journal of Historical Learning, Teaching and Research* 4: 67–106. [CrossRef]
Lincoln, Yvonna, and Egon Guba. 2000. The only generalization is: There is no generalization. In *Case Study Method*. Edited by Roger Gomm, Martyn Hammersley and Peter Foster. London: Sage.
Megill, Allan. 1994. Jorn Rusen's theory of historiography between modernism and rhetoric inquiry. *History and Theory* 33: 39–60. [CrossRef]
Merriam, Sharan. 1998. *Qualitative Research and Case Study Applications in Education*. San Francisco: Jossey-Bass.
Phillips, Mark. 2011. Rethinking historical distance: From doctrine to heuristic. *History and Theory* 50: 11–23. [CrossRef]
Rüsen, Jorn. 1993. The development of narrative competence in historical learning: An ontogenetic hypothesis concerning moral consciousness. In *Studies in Metahistory*. Edited by Jorn Rüsen. Pretoria: Human Sciences Council.
Rüsen, Jorn. 1996. Some theoretical approaches to intercultural comparative historiography. *History and Theory* 35: 5–22. [CrossRef]
Rüsen, Jorn. 2004. Historical consciousness: Narrative structure, moral function, and ontogenetic development. In *Theorizing Historical Consciousness*. Edited by Peter Seixas. Toronto: University of Toronto Press, pp. 63–85.
Rüsen, Jorn. 2006. Preface to the series. In *Narration, Identity and Historical Consciousness*. Edited by Jürgen Straub. New York: Berghahn Books.

Sandelowski, Margarete. 1995. Focus on qualitative methods, sample size in qualitative research. *Research in Nursing and Health* 18: 179–83. [CrossRef] [PubMed]

Santos, Carla, and Grace Yan. 2009. Genealogical tourism: A phenomenological examination. *Journal of Travel Research* 49: 56–67. [CrossRef]

Seixas, Peter. 2006. What is historical consciousness? In *To the Past: History Education, Public Memory, and Citizenship in Canada*. Edited by Ruth Sandwell. Toronto: Toronto University Press, pp. 11–22.

Shaw, Emma. 2020. "Who we are and why we do it": A demographic overview and the cited motivations of Australia's family historians. *Journal of Family History* 45: 109–24. [CrossRef]

Stake, Robert. 1995. *The Art of Case Study Research*. Los Angeles: Sage.

Tellis, Winston. 1997. Introduction to Case Study. *The Qualitative Report*. Available online: http://citeseerx.ist.psu.edu/viewdoc/download?doi=10.1.1.604.599&rep=rep1&type=pdf (accessed on 26 September 2021).

Thorpe, Robert. 2014. Towards an epistemological theory of historical consciousness. *Historical Encounters* 1: 17–28.

Yin, Robert. 1989. *Case Study Research: Design and Methods*. Thousand Oaks: Sage Publications.

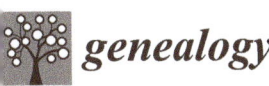

Article

Family Histories, Family Stories and Family Secrets: Late Discoveries of Being Adopted

Gary Clapton

Social Work Department, University of Edinburgh, Edinburgh EH8 9LD, UK; gary.clapton@ed.ac.uk

Abstract: This paper reviews what we know about the experiences of adopted people who discover in later-life that they are adopted. It begins by discussing how and why various facets of the adoption experience have come to the fore over the 20th and 21st century time span of contemporary adoption. The paper concludes with the fact that research on the late discovery of adoption is in its infancy. It also points to parallels that will exist for people who have been conceived by anonymous donation and raises additional areas for possible research.

Keywords: adoption; late-discovery; family secrets; shock and losses

Citation: Clapton, Gary. 2021. Family Histories, Family Stories and Family Secrets: Late Discoveries of Being Adopted. *Genealogy* 5: 105. https://doi.org/10.3390/genealogy5040105

Received: 9 November 2021
Accepted: 3 December 2021
Published: 8 December 2021

Publisher's Note: MDPI stays neutral with regard to jurisdictional claims in published maps and institutional affiliations.

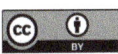

Copyright: © 2021 by the author. Licensee MDPI, Basel, Switzerland. This article is an open access article distributed under the terms and conditions of the Creative Commons Attribution (CC BY) license (https://creativecommons.org/licenses/by/4.0/).

1. Introduction

Any critical review of the history of modern adoption (that is, 20th and 21st adoption) would have to point out that the gaze of curiosity, professional attention and research has lighted upon different people and practices at different times. Broadly speaking, in the decades after legislation formalised adoption across much of the Anglophone nations, the focus was upon couples who wished to adopt and subsequently were setting out on adoptive parenthood. Knight's (1941) paper, 'Some Problems in Selecting and Rearing Adopted Children' is one example. In the 1950s, once adoptive families had been constituted and parenting adopted children had begun to present unique challenges, the focus became the adopted child and relations within his or her adoptive family (Barbara Raleigh begins her 1954 paper: 'David, age six, is an adopted child and a troubled child' (Raleigh 1954, p. 53)). Later, as adopted children entered adolescence and problems filtered through from practitioners, research interest grew in this field. In his well-known work on genealogical bewilderment, Sants wrote of 'A characteristic of the genealogically bewildered, particularly from adolescence onwards, is their relentless pursuit of the facts of their origin' (Sants 1964, p. 139).

From the 1970s onwards, the adult experiences of these children of the adoptions of 1940s and 1950s began to find their way into conferences, writings and books.[1] Special attention to searching and contact with birth families was prominent, and works appeared entitled, for example, *The Search for Anna* Fisher (1973) and *A Time to Search: The Moving and Dramatic Stories of Adoptees in Search of Their Natural* Parents (1977).[2] In the same broad chronological period, the birth mothers whose children were adopted in the 1940s and 1950s began to find their voices: *Birthmark* and *Death by Adoption* both came out in 1979 and are just two that heralded the opening of a floodgate of birth mother's accounts.

A rise in interest in reunions between adopted people and birth mothers in the 1990s corresponded with the alignment of the years of the highest number of adoptions in the UK (late 1960s) and that of the ages of adopted people most likely to seek contact—their late twenties (Clapton 1996).

Very broad brush, it is understood. Yet, over the last 70 years of adoption as we know it, attention to people and events in adoption seems to wax and wane connected to internal dynamics such as the age and capacity when adopted people are able to publicly express their experiences and when a birth mother can find her voice and get it into print but also, as indicated, external social factors—the 'boom' years of baby adoptions (the late 1960s) can be connected to a period 20 years later when interest began to grow and attention was paid to meetings between the children (now adult) and their birth parents. However, more simply, life span events, e.g., there was relatively little attention to adopted **adults** in the early years of modern adoption, instead, as indicated above, writings on adjusting to being an adoptive parent and raising an adoptive child can be associated with a growth 15 years later in attention to the problems of adolescents who are adopted. Certainly today, when most children are adopted from state care, it can be seen that much of the broad adoption discourse is taken up with engaging with the struggles of these children and their adoptive families. This somewhat impressionistic view of attentions and gazes in adoption should also note the temporary coming into focus of others such as birth fathers and other birth relatives such as brothers and sisters, and events and processes such as the long-term outcomes of reunions between adopted adults and their birth parents.[3]

Any critical history will always be subjective and selective. Some phases and periods overlap. There will be precursors. For example, McWhinnie was researching and writing on the experiences of adopted adults in the late 1950s. Her successful 1960 doctoral thesis was entitled *A Study of adoption: The Social Circumstances and Adjustment in Adult Life of 58 adopted children* (https://www.ed.ac.uk/alumni/services/notable-alumni/alumni-in-history/alexina-mcwhinnie (accessed on 31 October 2021)). Individual choice has featured in compiling this paper. Pelz notes, 'The logic of narration is more fictional than scientific' (Pelz 1990, p. 765), and so it will be for any history of adoption especially one that sets out to be critical. However, this is not the subject of this paper, but in the author's opinion, a necessary introduction to the main topic, the late discovery of being adopted. In 2009, Riley noted the lack of attention to late discovery, and since then there has been an increase in professional and academic attention (see below) together with the emergence of support networks such as Facebook groups. Https://en-gb.facebook.com/groups/latediscoveries/ (accessed on 31 October 2021) founded in 2011 is just one example. The secrecy that is baked into adoption, in a sense, is a 'gift' that keeps on giving. Down through the decades, the various struggles and challenges (and the pain) that have been touched on above are the fruits of subterfuge, denial and coverup. Whilst always having been a feature of the lives of adopted people, the **issue** of the late discovery of adoption is just one of the more recent of an accumulating legion of the challenges thrown up by myth and secrecy in adoption. Does the emergent research help us come to grips with this?

2. "If They Can Keep This a Secret from Me, What Else Are They Not Telling Me?"

Most of the writings on late discovery are personal experiences of adopted people, too many to enumerate here except to say that entering "late discovery adoptee" as a search term brings up over 7000 media stories, dedicated websites and support group forums and individual accounts, some in journals, others as stand alone.[4] 'One woman's story of the trauma of discovering at midlife that she'd been adopted' https://severancemag.com/a-dna-test-revealed-im-a-late-discovery-adoptee/ (2020) (accessed on 31 October 2021) is not untypical. Research papers that deal **directly** with the subject are much less in evidence, indeed, just three papers and a report could be found using the search phrase 'late discovery' combined with 'adopted adult', 'adoptee'. The first is that of Perl (2000), which consists of a telephone and in-person interview with 40 adopted people. Riley's work, also with Australian adult adoptees, (Riley 2008, 2009, 2013) consists of the analysis of 22 accounts of late discovery of adoption. The third, to date the more extensive paper, is that of Baden et al. (2019) and involved a survey of 254 adopted adults, nearly half of whom had found out about their adoption after the age of 11, with 92 finding out after turning 21 years old (one informant found out about their adoption when they were 78 yrs. old). A fourth publication of note is the Australian Government's report into a study of past adoption practices. Eight hundred and twenty-three adopted people took part in the quantitative phase of this study. Ninety-four respondents (11%) did not find out they had been adopted until they were 21 years of age or older. A further 70 adopted people found out between the ages of 11 and 20 years old (Kenny et al. 2012).

The paucity of the knowledge basis means that, undoubtedly, there is more to be said about the experiences and feelings of those who late-discover they have been adopted, however, five key themes and one issue appear in the existing literature. The issue in question is that of the **number** of people affected.

3. How Many Might Be Affected by the Late Discovery That They Are Adopted?

Based upon Riley's finding that 11% of her study of adopted adults had discovered in later life that they were adopted and on an estimate of 5 million adopted people in the USA, Baden et al. calculated that '550,000 U.S. adoptees, likely experienced delayed adoption disclosure or even nondisclosure altogether' (Baden et al. 2019, p. 1157). If Mignot's calculations relating to Western Europe (Mignot 2017) are used, then between 1900 and 2021, there have been 19,000 adoptions. Using the proportion of 11% as a guide, it would seem then that for this period, in Western Europe, over 200,000 people may have experienced late news of their adoption or none at all.[5] Given that Mignot's figures date from 1900, it will be likely that there will be less than 200,000 such adopted people alive now, however, their descendants will be, and as will be suggested, the ripples from late discovery can be extensive. However, let us now return to the event of late discovery itself. The following five themes of shock, betrayal, realisation of denial of difference, losses and legacies are derived from Riley (2008, 2009, 2013) and Baden et al. (2019) and in no hierarchical order. Though it seems right to begin with the event of the discovery.

4. Shock of Discovery

Riley comments that 'Late discoverers find out the truth of their origins in myriad ways. They find out by accident, are told by strangers, informed begrudgingly by family due to external pressures, and/or to cause pain or with insensitivity' (Riley 2013, p. 5). One of the informants in the Australian study by Kenny et al. testified thus:

> "When I found out I was adopted, it came completely out of the blue as a note on a birthday card sent from an aunt [by marriage], telling me that although I was adopted, I would always be her nephew. From this point, my life was shattered; the life I had been living up till now was a complete lie". (Kenny et al. 2012, p. 90)

At the same time as the shock, there is the additional feeling that everyone else knew of their adopted status except them: 'Barbara' (quoted in Riley) ' ... was 27 years old, and five months pregnant, when her mother admitted to her adoption during an ironing session' and she is quoted:

> " ... Yes, local shop-keepers, neighbours, school friends and just about anyone who knew us was aware of this 'secret'". (Riley 2013, p. 5)

Another prominent contemporaneous emotion is that of having been deceived.

5. Betrayal

Finding out adoptive status 'accidentally or from a stranger merely adds a further dimension of perceived betrayal to an already fraught emotional situation' (Riley 2013, p. 5). One of Riley's informants in an earlier study spoke of being " ... the brunt of a 40 year joke" ('Karla', in Riley 2009, p. 152). Two of the informants in one of the other Australian studies spoke of the discovery as meaning 'that my entire life up to the age of 49 was a lie' (Kenny et al. 2012, p. 90) and 'Devastated. My whole life was a lie. I never got over it' (Kenny et al. 2012, p. 90). The theme of deceit reaches back not just many years but in a perverse manner helps explain hitherto puzzling undercurrents in family dynamics.

6. The Conspiracy of Silence and Denial of Difference—Yet Unsurprised

Riley found that many were not surprised by the news of their adoption. The majority of the adopted people in her study reported that they had never felt they fitted in their families:

Most had usually looked different from the rest of their families, and had always felt that they were different in other ways, as well. Being told that they were adopted only confirmed pre-existing feelings and intuitions of being "other". (Riley 2013, p. 10)

Though unsurprised by the news, the task of comprehending the depth of dishonesty and lack of integrity and responsibility that has gone on through childhood, adolescence and adulthood is considerable and undoubtedly a contribution to the immediate distress at the point of late discovery. If there is any mitigating factor, there may be some relief from knowing that feelings of being the odd one out, the awkwardness felt at family gatherings and the evasions experienced when questions of family roots and histories arose can now be explained. These discomforts were not the fault of the adopted person.

Whilst feelings of shock and betrayal and distress over the extent of deceit may become less keen, there are some major losses that are not so diluted.

7. Losses: Kinship Confusion

In her study of Scottish adopted people and kinship, Carsten observes that:

The constitutive power of new kinship knowledge might be reinforced when such knowledge has been concealed. And this is because identity for Euro-Americans rests not just with self- knowledge, and hence kinship knowledge, but also with a sense of control over one's own life. (Carsten 2007, pp. 421–22).

In other words, knowledge of one's roots is essential to feel 'whole'. For those who discover they are adopted, this 'anchoring' sense of kinship is erased with all the turmoil and confusion that can be imagined from that.

Of those adopted people in her study, Perl noted that 'Some of the sample also experienced feelings of loss that their family was not their biological family, and questions of "who am I?" overwhelmed them' (Perl 2000, p. 3), and one of Kenny et al.'s informants: " ... felt I did not belong and was constantly confused about the way I was treated by my parents" (Kenny et al. 2012, p. 99). The third of the Australian studies on late-discoveries points out that those who experience this 'Not only do they have the family they grew up with, there is now another family 'out there', consisting of biological kin they know nothing about' (Riley 2013, p. 7). In Riley's earlier work, she quotes 'Zoe's' sorrow that finding out about her adoption in her forties left:

" ... little time to try to find any birth parents ... I did manage to meet my birth mother, and two sisters, but it was all too late. My birth mother was very old and sick ... incoherent ... and my birth sisters had had seriously sad and difficult lives". (Riley 2009, p. 153)

This is followed closely by Ursula's account of feeling adrift: " ... the most serious injustice afforded to me by late disclosure is that it prevented me from meeting my father and other members of my paternal family and developing a meaningful relationship with them during his lifetime" (Riley 2009, p. 153). This leads us to the next aspect of loss, agency.

8. Losses: Agency

The late discovery of adoption forces, produces and brings to the surface deep-seated identity questions. Perl talks of a grieving 'for the person whom one thought one was' (Perl 2000, p. 5). Kenny et al.'s informants echo this experience of loss of self: "It was as if my history was no longer mine ... ", and "Shocked, disbelieving, foolish, sense of self identity shattered". (Kenny et al. 2012, p. 90); a later informant in the same study was more blunt: "Upon disclosure, a big black hole opened up for me—"Who was I really?"" (Kenny et al. 2012, p. 99).

Riley suggests that those who discover their adopted then feel that ' ... they have had a 'false' identity imposed upon them; that they could have and probably would have grown and developed differently if they had been in possession of this knowledge about themselves ... ' (Riley 2013, p. 9).

9. Losses: Culture

Whilst all of us have cultures into which we are born and from which we come, for some of those who discover they are adopted, there can be broader range of consequences and complexity of losses. In Riley's study, 'Markus' discovered he was of aboriginal heritage: "I had fair skin and didn't know I was of Aboriginal descent" (Riley 2013, p. 9). Riley goes on to observe that the complexity of his discovery demanded an even greater intensity of re-orientation of his worldview and sense of self than others who did not have such specific cultural and ethnical bio-familial roots. This meant that alongside the decisions and tasks with which other late-discovery people had to engage such as learning about and searching for biological kin, this, for 'Markus', also encompassed 'learning about a new culture, a history of oppression ... ' and the systemic indignities to which his people had suffered (Riley 2013, p. 9).

Losses for late-discovery people can also be practical.

10. Losses: Medical History

Consider the chasm of health and medical and genetic knowledge that suddenly opens up on late discovery that the blood line that you thought you had was a fiction. This is closely coupled with the realisation that 'out there' there is another repository of information that is yours—but only if you can source it. 'Tina', one of Riley's informants, " ... found there was a history of mental illness in my natural family". She goes on, "Another thing I found out which really devastated me was there was a severe hearing problem in my family and I needed hearing aids immediately at the age of 33" (Riley 2013, p. 8).

Betrayed, conspired against and suffering multiple losses that range from the existential to vital practical health information. Add the fact that all of this might be experienced, felt, sensed and inflicted in seconds. If one can speak of an aftermath and consequences of late discovery, what might be a feature of the subsequent lives of these adopted people?

11. Legacies

Baden et al. suggest that experiences of late discovery have long-term consequences for relationships with others. Such experiences ' ... have the power to create ... interpersonal conflicts with others due to mistrust and other negative emotions and quote one informant who was aged 49 at the age of discovery':

"Realizing that you don't know who you are is life changing. Every relationship in my life changed at that moment. I am much more guarded in every aspect now. Finding out that everyone knew and I didn't is probably the single most traumatic event in my life". (Baden et al. 2019, p. 1171)

Baden et al. also draw attention to intrapersonal effects such as psychological distress: 'The adult adoptees in this study reported that learning of their adoption status as adults was significantly related to increased psychological distress even when measured many years after the adoption disclosure' (Baden et al. 2019, p. 1172).

12. Final Observations

Clearly, research on the experiences of the late discovery of adoptive status is in its infancy, certainly compared to the extent of Internet activity on the subject. What we can derive from the few existing works is that the late discovery of adoption can be considerably negatively significant for that adopted person's well-being and social relationships, and that late-discovery has long-term and lasting detrimental effects.

The obvious parallel with the experiences of people who discover they are adopted is that of those who have been conceived by donor. Riley (2013) and Baden et al. (2019)

make this connection. Our knowledge that considerably more donor-conceived adults have their status concealed from them than adopted adults (Daniels et al. 2009) means that further down the line, notwithstanding the international trends for the reversal of donor anonymity (Blyth and Frith 2013), sooner rather than later, there will be a similar burgeoning of research relating to the experiences of late-discovery of origins in this group of people.

Understandably there are gaps in the literature. Yet to be examined are the effects of late-discovery on others. The literature tends to treat those affected as atomised individuals, that is, adults without children (or grandchildren) or partners. We have yet to understand the effects on the lives of others close to an adopted person of late discovery. Indeed, what if the descendants of a deceased adopted person make the late discovery? DNA websites and services make this increasingly likely. Baden et al. (2019) observe that perhaps the later in life that one learns of her/his adoptive status the better because greater maturity can bring better coping skills—as compared with someone who learns that they are adopted when they are in their late teens. However, what about the timing and event-specific contexts of these discoveries? That is not just late in adult life compared with early adulthood, but how does late discovery effect, for example, someone undergoing a bereavement? Or a wedding? Or the birth of their child? One imagines, yes, of course, in all three examples, but that said, just how? On the one hand, there may be only so much a person can endure, mature adult or not, before they entertain darker thoughts of life's injustices. On the other hand, what of the pleasure that can be ushered in at a birth (or wedding)—what is to become of this when a late discovery lands on top of it? Finally, how late-discovery of being adopted differently affects men and women awaits research.

These gaps aside, it is clear from what we know already that whilst family histories are complex at the best of times, the late discovery of being adopted compounds this a thousand-fold.

Funding: This research received no external funding.

Institutional Review Board Statement: Not applicable.

Informed Consent Statement: Not applicable.

Data Availability Statement: Not applicable.

Conflicts of Interest: The author declares no conflict of interest.

Notes

[1] Studying trends in adoption as reflected in films will have to wait for another paper.

[2] This is not to say that prior to the 1970s adult adoptees were not visible in the discourses around adoption, see, for example, (Paton 1954).

[3] Other social factors that stand out once the span of adoption is considered include the rise of inter-country adoption, for example, as a result of a relative decline in the availability of white babies in the USA, adoptions of South Korean children increased from the 1970s. These adoptions in turn have produced the kind of fluctuating attention described here. For example, South Korea was the highest ranking country sending children for adoption overseas in the years 1980–1989 (Selman 2009). Once these children began to reach adulthood and articulate their experiences, the pace of public attention increased (Nelson et al. 2007). This is not to say that earlier experiences of Korean adoptees have not found their way into print. Jane Trenka was born in 1972, and her 2003 memoir of growing up adopted in rural Minnesota is widely acclaimed (Trenka 2003).

[4] The term 'late discovery adoptee' seems to have been coined by Morgan in the mid-1990s. His blog post (written under his name BB Church) provides a summary of the genesis of interest in the subject: http://bbchurch.blogspot.com/2006/05/ (accessed 31 October 2021).

[5] In Mignot's paper, 'Western Europe' is restricted to Germany, Sweden, France, England and Wales and Italy. Furthermore, given that the most recent decades have seen a major decline in the adoptions of babies (and a rise in adoptions of older children, holmanand not be subject to the kind of late-discovery experiences undergone by older adopted people. The percentage of 11% ought to thus be taken as broad guide rather than precise application because the percentage of late-discoveries will be less for adopted people under 30 years old and more for those over this age.

References

Baden, Amanda, Doug Shadel, Ron Morgan, Ebony White, Elliotte Harrington, Nicole Christian, and Todd Bates. 2019. Delaying Adoption Disclosure: A Survey of Late Discovery Adoptees. *Journal of Family Issues* 40: 1154–80. [CrossRef]
Blyth, Eric, and Lucy Frith. 2013. International Policy Trends Surrounding Donor Anonymity and Disclosure of Donor-Conceived Status. In Donor Conception: Lessons for Clinicians, Families, Policy Makers and Researchers, 20–21 June 2013, Montreal, Canada. (Unpublished). Available online: http://eprints.hud.ac.uk/id/eprint/18518/ (accessed on 31 October 2021).
Carsten, Janet. 2007. Connections and Disconnections of Memory and Kinship in Narratives of Adoption Reunions in Scotland. In *Ghosts of Memory: Essays on Remembrance and Relatedness*. Edited by Janet Carsten. Oxford: Blackwell.
Clapton, Gary. 1996. No more secrets and lies. *Community Care*, November 7, p. 27.
Daniels, Ken, Wayne Gillett, and Victoria Grace. 2009. Parental Information sharing with donor insemination conceived offspring: A follow-up study. *Human Reproduction* 24: 1099–105. [CrossRef] [PubMed]
Fisher, Florence. 1973. *The Search for Anna Fisher*. New York: A. Fields Books.
Kenny, Pauline, Daryl Higgins, Carol Soloff, and Reem Sweid. 2012. *Past Adoption Experiences: National Research Study on the Service Response to Past Adoption Practices*; Melbourne: Australian Institute of Family Studies.
Knight, Robert. 1941. Some Problems in Selecting and Rearing Adopted Children. *Bulletin of the Menninger Clinic* 5: 65–74.
Mignot, Jean-François. 2017. Full adoption in England and Wales and France: A comparative history of law and practice (1926–2015). *Adoption & Fostering* 41: 142–58.
Nelson, Kim Park, Elena Kim, and Leyne Myong Petersen. 2007. Proceedings of the First International Korean Adoption Studies Research Symposium. Dongguk University, Seoul, South Korea. Available online: http://kimparknelson.org/wp-content/uploads/2016/02/ikaa-final-2.pdf (accessed on 31 October 2021).
Paton, Jean. 1954. *The Adopted Break Silence: Forty Men and Women Describe Their Search for Natural Parents*. Philadelphia: Life History Study Center.
Pelz, Stephen. 1990. On systematic explanation in international history. *International History Review* 12: 762–78. [CrossRef]
Perl, Lynne. 2000. Why wasn't I told? Making sense of the late discovery of adoption. The Benevolent Society of New South Wales: Paddington, NSW Australia. Available online: https://www.americanadoptioncongress.org/docs/801%20-%20why-wasnt-i-told-may2001.pdf (accessed on 20 October 2021).
Raleigh, Barbara. 1954. Adoption as a factor in child guidance. *Smith College Studies in Social Work* 25: 53–71. [CrossRef]
Riley, Helen. 2008. The late discovery of adoptive status. *Family Relationships Quarterly* 7: 13–15.
Riley, Helen. 2009. Listening to late discovery adoption and donor offspring stories: Adoption, ethics and implications for contemporary donor insemination practices. In *Other People's Children: Adoption in Australia*. Edited by C. Spark and D. Cuthbert. Melbourne: Australian Scholarly Publishing, pp. 145–60.
Riley, Helen. 2013. Confronting the conspiracy of silence and denial of difference for late discovery adoptive persons and donor conceived people. *Australian Journal of Adoption* 7: 1–13.
Sants, Harriet. 1964. Genealogical bewilderment in children with substitute parents. *British Journal of Medical Psychology* 37: 133–40. [CrossRef] [PubMed]
Selman, Peter. 2009. The movement of children for international adoption: Developments and trends in receiving states and states of origin. 1998–2004. In *International Adoption: Global Inequalities and the Circulation of Children*. Edited by Diana Marre and Laura Briggs. New York: New York University Press, pp. 32–51.
Trenka, Jane. 2003. *The Language of Blood: A Memoir*. St Paul: Minnesota Historical Society Press.

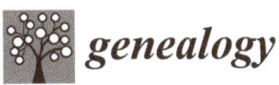

Review

Ancestral Selfies and Historical Traumas: Who Do You Feel You Are?

Pam Jarvis

Institute of Childhood and Education, Leeds Trinity University, Leeds LS18 5HD, UK; p.jarvis@leedstrinity.ac.uk

Abstract: The potential for 'historical trauma' is deeply rooted within the evolved human mind, which constructs its reality through narrative in the shape of personally and culturally relevant stories. From its roots within psychoanalytic theory and practice and through its clear links with infant attachment, historical trauma can be theoretically linked with stress biology and the concept of Adverse Childhood Experiences. Via this trajectory, it has the potential to become more commonly drawn upon in the field of public health, despite inconclusive attempts to link it to social epigenetics. It is proposed that when the historical trauma narrative invades family histories via negative experiences that have deeply impacted upon the lives of ancestors, descendants may be drawn to 'traumatic reenactment' through fantasy. This is explored with reference to my own recently published novel, examining its content through the perspective of the 'psychic work' it represents with respect to reconciling the self to the traumatic experiences of ancestors.

Keywords: historical trauma; traumatic reenactment; psychoanalysis; psychology; infant attachment; stress biology; Adverse Childhood Experiences

---

1. Introduction: The Story of the Story: Its Place in Human Lives

What place does storytelling hold in human life? This is a question I focused upon in a previous article for Genealogy "Not just *once* upon a time" (Jarvis 2019). In it, I extended a focus on narrative and storytelling with which I initially engaged during my PhD studies, over 20 years ago. My research at that time focused on young children's rough and tumble play, a phenomenon that had previously been overwhelmingly studied from a zoological and biological perspective. In my own investigations, the lens was turned towards ways in which young human beings bring storytelling into running, chasing, and play wrestling.

I found children adding comprehensive fantasies to chasing and catching play, drawn from concepts they had been introduced to both at home and at school, creatively translating underpinning narratives, such as fear, heroism, and salvation into original stories that were carried into their play, drawing upon a wide range of contemporary media heroes and events of the time (Jarvis 2007). This, I proposed, was because human beings have evolved as 'storying animals' living in a 'story-shaped world' (Lyle 2000, p. 55).

In my article for Genealogy I focused upon a sociological and cultural perspective.

'While stories are not living organisms, they are the cultural equivalent, the flexible carriers of the archetypal narrative, endlessly transformed by human beings to inform the next generation of universal 'truths' of what it is to be human, but within a vehicle that is continually culturally crafted to fit the listener.' Jarvis (2019, online)

At the time I was constructing 'Not just *once* upon a time' I was also starting to conceive a plan for a novel, drawn from ideas that had initially occurred to me during ancestry research on my own family. I had never seen or inherited any photographs or artefacts from my grandmother's father's family. The explanation she had given to me as a child was that of her father's early death and consequent geographical separation from her paternal

Citation: Jarvis, Pam. 2022. Ancestral Selfies and Historical Traumas: Who Do You Feel You Are? . *Genealogy* 6: 1. https://doi.org/10.3390/genealogy6010001

Received: 29 November 2021
Accepted: 21 December 2021
Published: 24 December 2021

Publisher's Note: MDPI stays neutral with regard to jurisdictional claims in published maps and institutional affiliations.

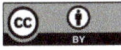

Copyright: © 2021 by the author. Licensee MDPI, Basel, Switzerland. This article is an open access article distributed under the terms and conditions of the Creative Commons Attribution (CC BY) license (https://creativecommons.org/licenses/by/4.0/).

grandparents. However, archival information I later retrieved indicated that this was not, in fact, the case.

When all the evidence was considered, it appeared that, following my great-grandfather's sudden death aged twenty-six, when my grandmother was only eighteen months old, there had been a disagreement between my grandmother's maternal and paternal grandparents and a consequent schism. I had previously idly mused when searching in historical archives for academic research that having a time portal would make the task much easier. I now had the same thought about the history of my own family.

Mulling over this issue brought a realization that, when the issue related to my own ancestors, it felt very different. A hypothetical question gradually emerged: so, what if I could travel in time to unravel the mystery, what would I do? The eventual product of this reflection was my first novel 'On Time' (Jarvis 2021) written over the 2020 pandemic lockdown. Creating this text involved drawing not only upon imagination to 'fill in the gaps' in the existing, incomplete family story that I had unearthed, but also upon my academic knowledge.

'On Time' focuses upon two women, both of whom, when suddenly confronted with the opportunity to travel in time, wrestle with temptation to 'fix' things in their ancestral past to prevent the occurrence of trauma that had impacted upon their ancestors. As I went through the process of exploring these ideas, particularly the trauma within 'Fran's' story, relating to oppressive religious and cultural beliefs that had impacted upon the lives of her grandmother and great-grandmother, I began to more deeply contemplate dynamics within my own ancestral family.

In building a cohesive story around this narrative, I became aware that I was now personally becoming involved in ancestral storytelling, an ancient pan-human activity I had previously explored in 'Not just once upon a time.' As I had also outlined in that article, I was engaging with this from my own cultural position within a media saturated, post-industrial society, framing the process in a contemporary, somewhat "mediated" manner, re-crafting Victorian events through my own twenty-first century lens, from the perspective of my own cultural 'truths' rather than those that had prevailed at the time.

Ancestry narratives are a fundamental example of the processes through which human brains create and recreate their reality through storying. But what 'psychic work' are we doing when we engage in this pursuit? The evidence suggests that motivations may be diverse, and emergent not only from conscious thought, but also from the unconscious.

2. My Ancestor, Myself: The Rise of the Historical Selfie

Nicholson (2018, p. 28) refers to ancestry research as a 'project of the self ... the story or narrative of who we are', comparing it to the social media 'selfie' photograph.

> 'Just as the selfie provides a self-portrait, possibly airbrushed, in the context of a person's temporal and geographical spaces, social networks and physical appearance, the genealogical project equally locates us in time, space, social status and physicality. They are both contemporary projects of the self—who we really think we are, aspire to be, and construct ourselves to be through the prism of how others act, exist, and have existed around us.' Nicholson (2018, p. 32).

While this may make ancestry research sound like a somewhat shallow and narcissistic pursuit, Lima (2019) posits that there are deeper psychological and sociological benefits in family history research for those who tell the stories, those who listen to them and the communities in which they are immersed. She proposes those who tell such stories are led to actively explore their identities and through so doing, may find increased psychic coherence; those who listen begin to realize that their story did not start from a blank slate at the beginning of their own life, and may become inspired by ancestors who have shown courage, particularly if they have survived against steep odds. Ancestral conversations lead people to engage in what Erikson (1950) referred to as 'generativity,' passing on wisdom to subsequent generations. Finally, communities may benefit from a sense of a shared past; a feeling that one is not such an isolated individual as it sometimes may seem. Kidron

(2003, p. 527) extends this agenda to a 'filial responsibility' to dead relatives, the process of keeping their voices alive: 'if we transmit their memories, the tree lives and if we don't it dies.' In summary, the stories of our ancestors animate the narrative of human descent; those who have lived and died before us spring to life once again in our imaginations.

However, there is an inherent danger in this process. As traditional stories develop over time, changing with the prevailing culture (Jarvis 2019), so family stories may also become lost and distorted within the march of time. Lents (2018) considers the benefits and detriments of becoming over-immersed in family history, citing the mass media influenced quest for a heroic and highly relatable story. He proposes that this leads to a tendency to think of distant ancestors, particularly those who lived in other parts of the world, as more similar to the self than would have in fact been possible. He also raises the enormous number of direct ancestors we have as we move beyond our great-grandparents, a fact that is sometimes forgotten in the impetus to seek out an illustrious ancestor who "belongs" to us. This is particularly prominent in some of the celebrity ancestry stories featured in British/American versions of the light entertainment show 'Who do you think you are,' where the search for royal or aristocratic ancestors may dominate (Holton and MacDonald 2019).

So, some of what we find in contemporary ancestry research, as in many fields of modern story telling is the 'commercializing and sanitizing' I previously explored in 'Not just *once* upon a time' (Jarvis 2019, online). In popular culture, the ancestry narrative can too easily be slickly 'storified' with the aim of creating good 'click-bait'; for example, a soap opera actor, a Prime Minister, an American film star, and a famous Olympian who have all descended from the same medieval king, without any mention of the fact that, by the law of statistics, a vast number of people with British ancestry will share the same ancient lineage (Lents 2018). However, there is an aspect of ancestry that underpins an arena of academic research and therapeutic methods within psychology: the devastating impact of historical trauma upon those whose ancestors' lives were shattered by tragedy.

3. Historical Trauma: Dissonant Echoes from the Past

While ancestry storytellers in popular media may sometimes be tempted to focus on telling an entertaining story of ancient royal and aristocratic ancestors in an hour of light entertainment, Kidron (2003, p. 15) raises the more intricate issue of 'trauma descendant identity,' proposing that where ancestors have experienced traumatic events, particularly early in life, the result may be that 'descendants ... suffer from maladaptive behavioral patterns and a damaged sense of self.' Her research explored psychological problems presented by people with ancestors who were survivors of tragic historical events such as the Holocaust and the Vietnam war, proposing that second and third generations can too easily become 'wounded descendants of historical trauma' (Kidron 2003, p. 532).

Sotero (2006) explores the origins of 'historical trauma theory', from its emergence in the 1960s, crafted from the notes of therapists working with families of Holocaust survivors, to its extension to other ethnic and national populations indirectly impacted by events that shattered the lives of ancestors. Examples include example war, slavery, and forced migrations, including those from Palestinian, African American, Vietnamese, Russian, Cambodian, Alaskan, and Native American heritages.

> 'Offspring of parents affected by trauma also exhibited various symptoms of PTSD or "historical trauma response." These symptoms included an array of psychological problems such as denial, depersonalization, isolation, memory loss, nightmares, psychic numbing, hypervigilance, substance abuse, fixation on trauma, identification with death, survivor guilt, and unresolved grief.' Sotero (2006, p. 96).

She adds a reflection upon the likelihood that the degree of trauma would depend to some extent upon the intent of the oppressors; for example, were their actions intended to elicit obedience to a group norm, or to silence people who espoused an opposing point of view, or at the most violent extreme, to murder whole populations from a particular nation or ethnicity?

Sotero (2006, p. 99) created an overview conceptual model of historical trauma. See Figure 1 below.

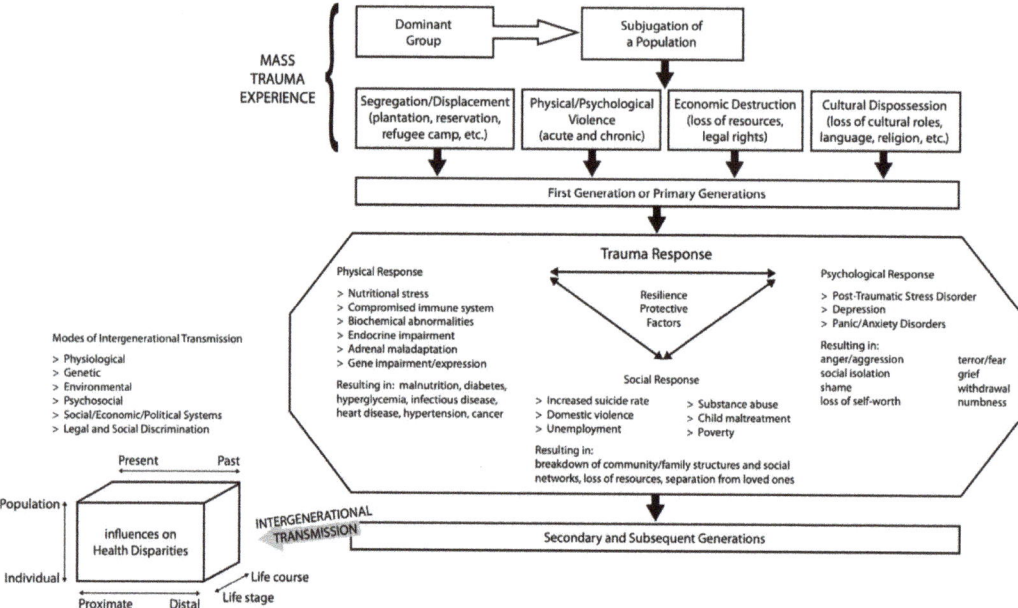

Figure 1. Conceptual model of historical trauma. Source: Sotero (2006, p. 99).

This issue is explored in 'On Time' (Jarvis 2021) in what is shared and not shared by three female protagonists of different ethnic heritage, 'Fran', 'Annamarie', and 'Suzi.' While Fran is convinced that her great-grandfather's early death condemned her grandmother to an unhappy childhood in a household immersed in oppressive religious and cultural beliefs, Annamarie becomes increasingly obsessed with the deep trauma her grandmother has suffered from the loss of her mother in the Holocaust, eventually seeking a way that this might be assuaged in the present, via the illicit use of a time portal.

When the characters discover Annamarie's actions, it falls to Suzi to explain, from her perspective as a second generation Vietnamese American, why Annamarie's situation is different to Fran's:

> 'Do you remember when you showed me your great-grandmother's china tea set, Fran? My family has nothing like that, nor will Annamarie's Grandma Rachel. All of these things left behind in the place they had to run from .... Neither Annamarie nor I even share a common first language with our great-grandparents ... So, Fran was tempted to rescue her great-grandfather because he died from what is now an easily curable illness. That's eminently understandable. But how tempted do you think you might be to pull your ancestor out of the inferno of the twentieth century, if you had that chance?' Jarvis (2021, pp. 90–91).

While Fran's ancestors have experienced the death of a young father and subsequently been oppressed by other family members who wish to force them to comply with punitive religious and cultural beliefs, part of Annamarie's ancestral family has been systematically murdered by a genocidal state. The opportunity to travel through time to rescue ancestral relatives is of course where fact ends and fantasy begins. However, the process of subsequent generations like Fran and Annamarie still seeking resolution for the suffering of their ancestors (Wardi 1992) is a very real phenomenon that has been extensively explored by psychological researchers and psychoanalysts.

'On Time' depicts Annamarie's mother, Linda, as being of a nervous disposition. It also transpires she has named Annamarie for her lost great-grandmother, Anna. Annamarie's grandmother Rachel frequently comments upon her resemblance to Anna: 'Sometimes, I think you get more and more like her, and other times, I think I am just telling a story; one that brings her back, somehow. I can't really remember her face or her voice anymore' (Jarvis 2021, p. 38). Children placed in such a position are forced into a role of 'memorial candle' (Wardi 1992).

The story of a family dominated by historical trauma is one that contains empty places that it yearns to fill; hence the temptation to construct the child as the member with the duty to fill it. But because the child can never be the same person as the lost relative, the process cannot create a satisfactory resolution for those who have been so traumatically bereaved.

Wardi (1992) describes a therapeutic interaction in which her client tells her that, while it might appear to others that her family has honored her by naming her for her father's sister, murdered in the Holocaust, in the end this occludes her relationship with her father.

> 'The father thus sees his sister in his daughter . . . and unconsciously transmits to her all the complexity of his unsolved feelings for her. But he doesn't see his daughter or any of what she feels, what she needs . . . the ambivalent position of the "memorial candles" in their parents' consciousness. In the face of the images of perished objects, who were idealized after death in the survivors' psyche, the "memorial candles" have no chance.' Wardi (1992, p. 37).

Wardi (1992, p. 11) also considers the fragmentary emotions of the survivors towards dead relatives that may then be projected onto the 'substitute.' One of her patients, a woman who, as a teenager, experienced her mother's murder on a Nazi death march, has unresolved feelings of abandonment and guilt. On the one hand, the mother abandoned the daughter by dying, but on the other, the daughter feels that she abandoned the mother: 'she allowed her to die alone at the side of the road and thus lost her own self as well.' Wardi concludes that 'memorial candles' are trapped in relationships where they are unable to claim an identity that is truly separate from the existing one that they have been allocated by the family; they become completely enmeshed in their family's tragedy.

The theme of enmeshment is picked up in 'On Time', where on being presented with the opportunity to travel in time, Fran initially intends to impartially observe her ancestral family's Victorian Presbyterianism, with a view to an increased understanding of the lives of her grandmother and great-grandmother. Once she enters their world, however, she becomes sorely tempted to interfere in the timeline to prevent what she sees as the trigger for the cascade of traumatic events that blighted her grandmother's childhood: the premature death of her great-grandfather. Annamarie becomes determined to orchestrate a macabre reunion between her grandmother and great-grandmother to assuage their loss of one another in events leading up to the Holocaust. Both women have over-identified with the abandonment their grandmothers experienced and both therefore set out to atone for this as 'wounded healers' (Benziman et al. 2012) on an impossible mission to mend lives that were shattered before they were born.

At this point, however, fiction leaves fact behind, because in real life those experiencing such trauma do not have access to a time portal! The typical trajectory of historical trauma therefore creates a build-up of repressed emotion within the unconscious minds of descendants, which seeps into consciousness as an unresolvable feeling of separation anxiety. Wolynn (2016) suggests that release may then be unconsciously pursued through a 'traumatic re-enactment' defense bubbling up into the subconscious which hangs stories upon the separation narrative via dreams and fantasies (Freud 1961).

It is interesting to speculate whether this process may lie at the heart of many novels, the unconscious of the author harnessing imagination and creativity to process feelings through the crafting of a story to hang upon the trauma narrative that stalks the dark corridors of their mind. Perhaps then, my own unconscious may have motivated me to create imaginary characters with historical traumas, thence to work further on this through a fantasy where they gain access to a time portal.

This was not a situation of which I was consciously aware in the planning or early writing stages. I had started the novel from the perspective of working through the loose ends in my ancestry story in a way that would allow me to tie them together more neatly; in this, I drew upon the historian parts of my mind, not initially realizing that a psychodynamic process was involved. It was only in retrospect that this emerged. My first reflection on my own psychological perspective as the author came from the fact that, when the story arc curtailed 'Fran's' travels in time, the theme did not feel fully closed to me until the character was depicted as writing her own novel, telling the anonymous story of her family, drawing upon her experience of meeting them via her journeys into the past. Even in this fiction then, my unconscious compelled me to tell not only the granddaughter's story, but also the grandmother's. It was from this thought that an inkling arose that historical trauma within my own psyche was playing a part in the authoring, not least because my grandmother had played such a significant and direct role in my childhood. For 'Annamarie', while the grandmother's story is told, the granddaughter's is as yet unfinished, and still bound up with the fate of the great-grandmother. This will be further worked upon in a sequel, with the author far more aware of the psychodynamic forces at play within the process.

In 2006, the actor Stephen Fry explored a historical trauma within his own family, in one of the most compelling and poignant episodes of the British 'Who do you think you are' series (BBC 2006), which engages with a story of historic trauma. When he began his research by talking to his parents about their family memories, he discovered that his mother, though born and raised in England, had an Austrian aunt and cousins, murdered in the Holocaust, whose 'ghosts' had deeply impacted upon her childhood. She recalled that her parents had been 'so upset' when they realized that she had discovered a photograph of these relatives, only reluctantly disclosing to her that 'they had all been killed', then refusing to discuss the matter further. The main trajectory of the program is Fry's quest to discover what happened to these lost relatives, in particular exactly when and where they had died.

This, then, is a less overt familial response to historical trauma than the creation of 'memorial candles', but one that may equally create emotional dysfunction in descendants. As Bar-On et al. (1998, p. 331) comment, a 'conspiracy of silence' cannot be total. Sooner or later, someone in the family will raise the issue, and then the imagination of the descendant may fill in the gaps, a situation in which I found myself when I realized that my grandmother had hidden part of her childhood from me.

In this sense then, the 'Fran' character in 'On Time' finds herself in the position of discovering a family-located trauma that has been hidden from her, whilst 'Annamarie' has been cast in the role of 'memorial candle' for a great-grandmother destroyed by genocide, which the story draws upon to explain her greater impetus to follow her 'rescue mission' to completion. It is unclear where 'Suzi' finds herself in this respect, but she demonstrates that she can access the overarching narrative of historical trauma, and consequently empathize with the feelings of both, clearly articulating the difference between the historical trauma stories that Fran and Annamarie's ancestors have bequeathed to them.

In summary, it is evident that those whose ancestors experienced traumatic events cannot easily avoid secondary impacts; both knowing and not knowing may equally become a source of historical trauma. 'Small details of the Holocaust experience may affect the second generation pervasively, just because only part of the story is being told and much is left to the imagination' Bar-On et al. (1998, p. 332). Historical trauma demonstrates the human reliance upon stories to shape our existence and provides evidence to indicate that this process can sometimes work against our well-being.

When the 'storying' concept is considered, it becomes clear that specific stories that are woven around the underlying narrative of human trauma by second generation survivors are typically underpinned by feelings of abandonment and loss. Wolynn (2016, p. 3) refers to the familial transmission of a 'personal language of fear', proposing that his family's trauma had been transmitted as a feeling of helplessness to him, where being stripped of identity and alone 'echoed traumas that took place in my family history before I was born.' To further explore this process, the theory of infant attachment and its extension into stress response biology must be explored.

4. The Role of Attachment in Historical Trauma

The concept of human infant attachment was created by the British psychologist John Bowlby over the period directly following World War II (1939–1945). Bowlby had a long-standing interest in the ethology of imprinting in avian species, and subsequently created his theory by mixing concepts from this research with insights gathered in his psychoanalytic work with children who had been evacuated or otherwise separated from their families during the war (Jarvis 2020). His central proposal was that, based on their earliest relationships, infants construct an 'Internal Working Model' (IWM) of what to expect from other people, and consequently of their own level of 'lovability'. He proposed that this was the basis of all subsequent emotional interactions with others, both in childhood and in later life: ''No concept within the attachment framework is more central to developmental psychiatry than that of the secure base' (Bowlby 1988, pp. 163–64).

Bowlby's associate Mary Ainsworth subsequently explored the quality of attachment that 18-month-old babies had to their mothers (Ainsworth 1967), finding that where infants experience their mothers as being emotionally available to them, they develop social and emotional confidence. But if an infant intuits that their mother is never or only conditionally emotionally available, they became socially and emotionally anxious. Wolynn (2016, p. 3) evokes how this has translated to adulthood for him; a constant underlying fear that he will be left alone to cope with his problems.

Bar-On et al. (1998, p. 318) describe a 'secondary traumatisation' effect in the offspring of trauma survivors, which 'presents some systematic evidence for transmission affects across two generations . . . attachment theory and its recent research advances provide an appropriate conceptual framework.' They cite the work of Van IJzendoorn (1995) who found that where parents of infants reported childhood experiences that had negatively impacted upon their emotional security and insecure attachment with their parents, this was highly correlated with insecure attachment patterns in their own young children.

Clearly, this process has the potential to become a generational cascade, and where grandparents are closely involved in the care of grandchildren there may also be the potential for direct transmission to two subsequent generations.

> 'Being left by a close attachment figure aroused feelings of anger even if the separation was caused by death. Many survivors still seem to maintain anger toward their parents because they were left alone. However, they have difficulty in overtly expressing this anger because of the tragic circumstances under which separation took place and they run the risk of being left with an unresolved mourning process . . . This orientation significantly deviates from what Bowlby believed to be so critical to the healthy development of infants . . . emotional accessibility which would lead to "felt security" on the part of the infant.' Bar-On et al. (1998, pp. 320–21).

Attachment theory is still very much a 'live' entity in the twenty first century, with the Internal Working Model at its heart. Over the past twenty years, it has been further validated by biological evidence, in which researchers have correlated variations in stress biology against levels of emotional security in infants. Patterns of abnormally raised levels of the stress hormone cortisol in young children can be reliably detected in situations where the care that they are receiving is fragmented and, from the child's perspective, uncertain.

> 'The core empirical evidence from nearly two decades of cortisol studies indicates that when children experience ongoing stress due to early insecure relationships with adults that destabilize their emotional equilibrium, this sets in train

a problem with stress management that may eventually become 'toxic' to that individual.' (Jarvis 2020, online).

This would seem to fit the emergence of historical trauma in families in which parents are impacted by traumatic events before the children were born. The anxiety created by these events does not evaporate but remains within the individual's psychological functioning, later impacting upon the relationships that they build with their own children, an effect Bar-On et al. (1998, p. 318) refer to as 'secondary traumatisation.' Furthermore, as insecure attachment patterns are highly likely to be passed from one generation to the next, it has the extended potential to create a cascade, in which subsequent generations of the family are impacted in turn.

Felitti et al. (1998) carried out research into physical and mental health impacts emergent from 'Adverse Childhood Experiences', exploring the long-term consequences of family dysfunction in the stress biology of a large sample of adults based in the US. They found overwhelming evidence of a strong correlation between traumatic childhood experiences, poor stress coping, cortisol dysfunction, and ongoing mental and physical health problems. What is now termed 'ACEs' research has extended across the world, making concordant findings.

Large-scale studies in England (Bellis et al. 2014), Wales (Bellis et al. 2015), and Scotland (Coupar and Mackie 2016) have linked cortisol disturbance, dysfunctional stress response, and poor mental/physical health in adulthood to childhood ACEs. Steele et al. (2016) extended the focus to an exploration of environmental stressors upon parents, and the markers that this creates in offspring stress biology. Historical trauma is a phenomenon that has clear potential to be added to this theoretical arena.

NHS Highland use the following figure (Figure 2) to illustrate the range of ACEs currently being explored by researchers, dividing them into Adverse Childhood Experiences and Adverse Community Experiences:

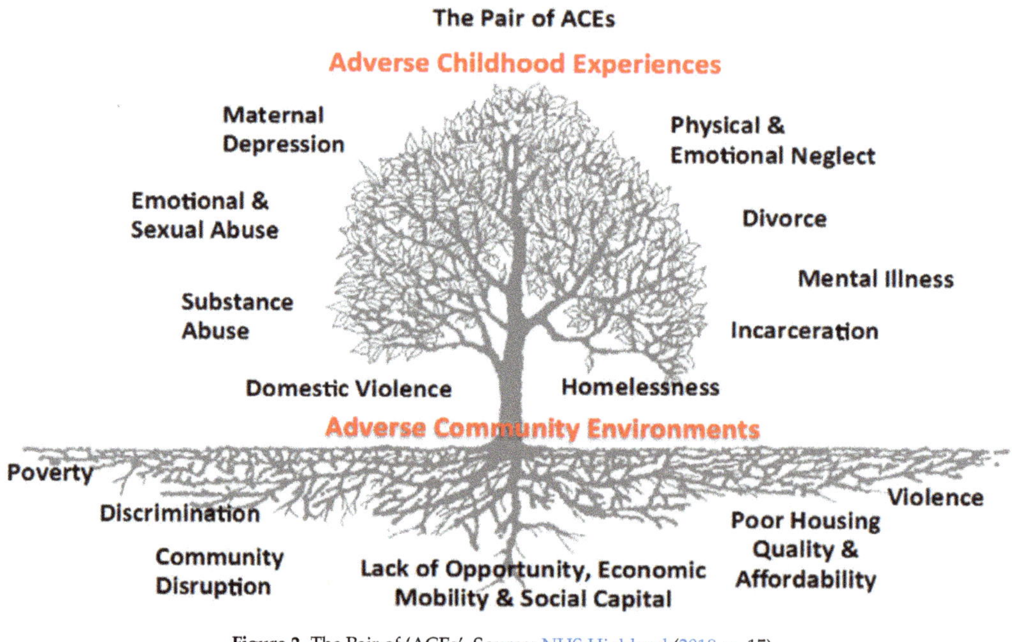

The Pair of ACEs

Adverse Childhood Experiences

- Maternal Depression
- Physical & Emotional Neglect
- Emotional & Sexual Abuse
- Divorce
- Mental Illness
- Substance Abuse
- Incarceration
- Domestic Violence
- Homelessness

Adverse Community Environments

- Poverty
- Violence
- Discrimination
- Poor Housing Quality & Affordability
- Community Disruption
- Lack of Opportunity, Economic Mobility & Social Capital

Figure 2. The Pair of 'ACEs'. Source: NHS Highland (2018, p. 15).

The concept of 'historical trauma' can therefore draw upon a wide body of research for future theoretical and empirical progression. As Sotero (2006, p. 102) proposes, it is becoming increasingly well placed to integrate into initiatives that 'help public health practitioners and researchers gain a broader perspective of health disparities and aid in the development of new approaches'.

However, one branch of historical trauma research has recently been immersed in controversy: a contested attempt to link it into the newly forged arena of Social Epigenetics.

5. Social Epigenetics: A Bridge Too Far?

Epigenetics is a relatively new branch of biology that explores the interaction of gene expression and environment. 'Gene expression refers to how often or when proteins are created from the instructions within your genes. While genetic changes can alter which protein is made, epigenetic changes affect gene expression to turn genes "on" and "off"'. (Center for Disease Control and Prevention 2020, online).

In the first decade of the 21st century, it was discovered that people who were fetuses in utero during the Dutch Hunger Winter of 1944–1945, but who were not significantly deprived of nourishment after birth carried specific epigenetic markers that they shared with one another, but not with their biological relatives. 'These data are the first to contribute empirical support for the hypothesis that early-life environmental conditions can cause epigenetic changes in humans that persist throughout life' (Heijmans et al. 2008, p. 17046).

Two years earlier, Sotero (2006) had raised the need to strengthen the validity of historical trauma theory with quantitative, empirical evidence. Historical trauma theory therefore enthusiastically picked up upon the prospect of epigenetic alteration in fetuses in utero, created by trauma previously experienced by their parents:

> 'Alteration(s) in offspring may be mediated by mental health symptoms during gestation, and certainly extend to the postnatal environment. In studies of Holocaust offspring, perhaps the most salient observation has been that most differences in offspring phenotype were associated with persistent psychological effects of parents.' Yehuda and Lehrner (2018, online).

What the authors are doing here is speculating that epigenetic changes might be a response not only to a physical trauma like starvation, but also to neurological changes in the parent created by stress, impacting upon the genetic heritage of the child. However, this is clearly difficult to support retrospectively as there is no clear beginning and end to anxiety in the way that there is to starvation. Any epigenetic changes in the second generation may therefore have occurred at any stage of life; it cannot be neatly tracked back to the gestational period.

The 'gestational effects' proposal was therefore swiftly refuted by the wider biological community, as an 'attractive but poorly-founded idea' (Center for Epigenomics at the Albert Einstein College of Medicine 2015, online). In an extensive literature review on epigenetics, Deichmann (2020, online) urges caution: 'since the idea of transgenerational inheritance of epigenetic marks has become fashionable, the temptation of epigenetic hype and the danger of lowering critical standards is prevalent.'

The proposal that historical trauma may be transmissible during gestation by gene altering environmental stress continues to intrigue, but is currently insufficiently supported by empirical research. However, research that has overwhelmingly supported the existence of biological impacts created by childhood stressors does indicate that there may be clear links with historical trauma. Historical trauma theory also has concordance with classical attachment theory and with the findings of the ACEs researchers. It is therefore highly likely that the concept of historical trauma could find a secure place within the theory and practice of 'ACEs,' and subsequently become a feature within mainstream public health initiatives.

6. Conclusions: The Future for Historical Trauma Theory

The links between ancestry research and child development may seem tenuous from a populist 'ancestry as selfie' perspective. However, viewed from the perspective of human beings as a 'storying animal' sharing abstract thoughts shaped by overarching narratives recounted within culturally relevant story forms, the links become more obvious. My own experience of drawing upon the historical trauma narrative through the crafting of a novel based on ancestral events serves as a useful example of 'traumatic reenactment' though fantasy, a phenomenon which may be a commonplace mechanism in creative human storying.

The concept of historical trauma is now well poised to move into mainstream psychology through its links to attachment theory and the swiftly developing theory and practice arena that explores the devastating effects of 'Adverse Childhood Experiences.' It also has the potential to further secure its place within this arena through ongoing biological research relating to the impacts of poorly calibrated stress biology upon mental and physical health. The fact that attempts to link historical trauma to social epigenetics have not currently been successful should not create a barrier to this progression.

In conclusion, the concept of historical trauma has a promising future as a theoretical lens that can deepen understanding of how it feels to inhabit a human, storying mind. Our emotional memories clearly encompass a past and a future that extends beyond the physical existence of the self, into the experiences of ancestors who are now dead, and those that will eventually unfold for descendants who are yet to be.

Funding: This research received no external funding.

Institutional Review Board Statement: Not applicable.

Informed Consent Statement: Not applicable.

Data Availability Statement: Not applicable.

Conflicts of Interest: The author declares no conflict of interest.

References

Ainsworth, Mary. 1967. *Infancy in Uganda: Infant Care and the Growth of Love*. Baltimore: Johns Hopkins University Press.

Bar-On, Dan, Jeanette Eland, Rolf. J. Kleber, Robert Krell, Yael Moore, Abraham Sagi, Erin Soriano, Peter Suedfeld, Peter G. van der Velden, and Marinus H. van IJzendoorn. 1998. Multigenerational Perspectives on Coping with the Holocaust Experience: An Attachment Perspective for Understanding the Developmental Sequelae of Trauma across Generations. *International Journal of Behavioral Development* 22: 315–38. Available online: https://psycnet.apa.org/record/1998-04280-005 (accessed on 26 November 2021).

BBC. 2006. Who Do You Think You Are [Series 2, Episode 3, Stephen Fry]. Available online: https://www.youtube.com/watch?v=6XajHxoCpXY (accessed on 26 November 2021).

Bellis, Mark A., Kathryn Ashton, Karen Hughes, Katharine Ford, Julie Bishop, and Shantini Paranjothy. 2015. *Adverse Childhood Experiences and Their Impact on Health-Harming Behaviours in the Welsh Adult Population*. Cardiff: Public Health Wales. Available online: http://www2.nphs.wales.nhs.uk:8080/PRIDDocs.nsf/7c21215d6d0c613e80256f490030c05a/d488a3852491bc1d80257f370038919e/$FILE/ACE%20Report%20FINAL%20(E).pdf (accessed on 26 November 2021).

Bellis, Mark A., Kathryn Hughes, Nicola Leckenby, Clare Perkins, and Helen Lowey. 2014. National household survey of adverse childhood experiences and their relationship with resilience to health-harming behaviors in England. *BMC Medicine* 12: 72. Available online: https://bmcmedicine.biomedcentral.com/articles/10.1186/1741-7015-12-72 (accessed on 26 November 2021). [CrossRef]

Benziman, Galia, Ruth Kannai, and Ayesha Ahmad. 2012. The Wounded Healer as Cultural Archetype. *CLCWeb: Comparative Literature and Culture* 14: 1. Available online: https://docs.lib.purdue.edu/cgi/viewcontent.cgi?article=1927&context=clcweb (accessed on 26 November 2021). [CrossRef]

Bowlby, John. 1988. *A Secure Base*. London: Routledge.

Center for Disease Control and Prevention. 2020. What Is Genetics? Available online: https://www.cdc.gov/genomics/disease/epigenetics.htm (accessed on 26 November 2021).

Center for Epigenomics at the Albert Einstein College of Medicine. 2015. Over-Interpreted Epigenetics Study of the Week. Available online: https://epgntxeinstein.tumblr.com/post/127416455028/over-interpreted-epigenetics-study-of-the-week (accessed on 26 November 2021).

Coupar, Sarah, and Phil Mackie. 2016. *Polishing the Diamonds: Addressing Adverse Childhood Experiences in Scotland*. Glasgow: Public Health Scotland. Available online: https://www.scotphn.net/wp-content/uploads/2016/06/2016_05_26-ACE-Report-Final-AF.pdf (accessed on 26 November 2021).

Deichmann, Ute. 2020. The Social Construction of the Social Epigenome and the Larger Biological Context. *Epigenetics & Chromatin* 13: 37. Available online: https://www.ncbi.nlm.nih.gov/pmc/articles/PMC7510271/ (accessed on 26 November 2021). [CrossRef]

Erikson, Erik. H. 1950. *Childhood and Society*. New York: Norton.
Felitti, Vincent, Robert Anda, Dale Nordenberg, David Williamson, Alison Spitz, Valerie Edwards, Mary Koss, and James Marks. 1998. Relationship of childhood abuse and household dysfunction to many of the leading causes of death in adults. *American Journal of Preventative Medicine* 14: 245–58. Available online: https://pubmed.ncbi.nlm.nih.gov/9635069/ (accessed on 26 November 2021). [CrossRef]
Freud, Sigmund. 1961. *Beyond the Pleasure Principle*. Translated by J. Strachey. New York: W. W. Norton and Company.
Heijmans, Bastiann T., Elmar W. Tobi, Aryeh D. Stein, Hein Putter, Gerard J. Blauw, Ezra. S. Susser, Eline P. Slagboom, and L. H. Lumey. 2008. Persistent epigenetic differences associated with prenatal exposure to famine in humans. *Proceedings of the National Academy of Sciences* 105: 17046–49. Available online: https://www.pnas.org/content/105/44/17046 (accessed on 26 November 2021). [CrossRef]
Holton, Graham, and Alisdair MacDonald. 2019. Danny Dyer Has Royal Ancestors—How Likely Is It You Do Too? The Conversation. Available online: https://theconversation.com/danny-dyer-has-royal-ancestors-how-likely-is-it-you-do-too-110227 (accessed on 26 November 2021).
Jarvis, Pam. 2007. Monsters, Magic and Mr. Psycho: Rough and Tumble Play in the Early Years of Primary School, a Biocultural Approach. *Early Years, An International Journal of Research and Development* 27: 171–88. Available online: https://www.tandfonline.com/doi/abs/10.1080/09575140701425324 (accessed on 26 November 2021).
Jarvis, Pam. 2019. Not Just 'Once' Upon a Time. *Genealogy* 3: 44. Available online: https://www.mdpi.com/2313-5778/3/3/44 (accessed on 26 November 2021). [CrossRef]
Jarvis, Pam. 2020. Attachment theory, Cortisol and Care for the under 3s in the 21st Century: Constructing evidence-informed policy. *Early Years, An International Journal of Research*. Available online: https://www.tandfonline.com/doi/full/10.1080/09575146.2020.1764507 (accessed on 26 November 2021).
Jarvis, Pam. 2021. *On Time*. Milton Keynes: Burton Meyers Books.
Kidron, Carol A. 2003. Surviving a Distant past: A Case Study of the Cultural Construction of Trauma Descendant Identity. *Ethos* 31: 513–44. Available online: https://psycnet.apa.org/record/2004-11595-003 (accessed on 26 November 2021).
Lents, Nathan. 2018. The Meaning and Meaninglessness of Genealogy: Researching our Family Background Is All the Rage, but What Does It All Mean? Available online: https://www.psychologytoday.com/gb/blog/beastly-behavior/201801/the-meaning-and-meaninglessness-genealogy (accessed on 26 November 2021).
Lima, Anna. 2019. Family History and Genealogy: The Benefits for the Listener, the Storyteller and the Community. *Journal of Cape Verdean Studies* 4: 63–74. Available online: https://vc.bridgew.edu/jcvs/vol4/iss1/ (accessed on 26 November 2021).
Lyle, Sue. 2000. Narrative Understanding: Developing a Theoretical Context for Understanding How Children Make Meaning in Classroom Settings. *Journal of Curriculum Studies* 32: 45–63. Available online: https://www.tandfonline.com/doi/abs/10.1080/002202700182844 (accessed on 26 November 2021).
NHS Highland. 2018. Adverse Childhood Experiences, Resilience and Trauma Informed Care: A Public Health Approach to Understanding and Responding to Adversity. Available online: https://www.nhshighland.scot.nhs.uk/Publications/Documents/DPH-Annual-Report-2018_(web-version).pdf (accessed on 26 November 2021).
Nicholson, Paula. 2018. Family Trees, Selfies and our search for Identity. *The Psychologist* 31: 28–32. Available online: https://thepsychologist.bps.org.uk/volume-31/november-2018/family-trees-selfies-and-our-search-identity (accessed on 26 November 2021).
Sotero, Michelle. 2006. A Conceptual Model of Historical Trauma: Implications for Public Health Practice and Research. *Journal of Health Disparities Research and Practice* 1: 93–108. Available online: http://www.ressources-actuarielles.net/EXT/ISFA/1226.nsf/9c8e3fd4d8874d60c1257052003eced6/bbd469e12b2d9eb2c12576000032b289/$FILE/Sotero_2006.pdf (accessed on 26 November 2021).
Steele, Howard, Jordan Bate, Miriam Steele, Shanta Rishi Dube, Kerri Danskin, Hannah Knafo, Adella Nikitiades, Karen Bonuk, Paul Meissner, and Anne Murphy. 2016. Adverse Childhood Experiences, poverty and parenting stress. *Canadian Journal of Behavioural Science* 48: 32–38. Available online: https://psycnet.apa.org/record/2016-01736-004 (accessed on 26 November 2021).
Van IJzendoorn, Marinus H. 1995. Adult attachment representations, parental responsiveness, and infant attachment: A meta-analysis on the predictive validity of the Adult Attachment Interview. *Psychological Bulletin* 117: 387–403. Available online: https://pubmed.ncbi.nlm.nih.gov/7777645/ (accessed on 26 November 2021).
Wardi, Dina. 1992. *Memorial Candles: Children of the Holocaust*. London: Routledge.
Wolynn, Mark. 2016. *It Didn't Start with You: How Inherited Family Trauma Shapes Who We Are and How to End the Cycle*. New York: Penguin.
Yehuda, Rachel, and Amy Lehrner. 2018. Intergenerational transmission of trauma effects: Putative role of epigenetic mechanisms. *World Psychiatry: Official Journal of the World Psychiatric Association (WPA)* 17: 243–57. Available online: https://www.ncbi.nlm.nih.gov/pmc/articles/PMC6127768/ (accessed on 26 November 2021). [CrossRef]

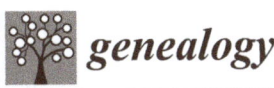

Article

How Key Psychological Theories Can Enrich Our Understanding of Our Ancestors and Help Improve Mental Health for Present and Future Generations: A Family Historian's Perspective

Helen Parker-Drabble

Independent Researcher, London W1A 6US, UK; helen@helenparkerdrabble.com or h_parker_drabble@hotmail.com; Tel.: +44-7871-203-644

Abstract: Family historians could increase their understanding of their ancestors and themselves and improve the mental health of living and future generations if they consider the psychological history of their forebears. Genealogists could then begin to recognize their family's unique psychological inheritance that can appear as a result of trauma, depression, or addiction. The author explores three generations of a Parker family branch from Huntingdon/Norfolk, England, to show family historians how such considerations can shed light on their family's psychological legacy. The author does this by introducing us to her great-grandmother Ann grandfather Walter, and mother Doreen through the lens of attachment theory, and their adverse childhood experiences (ACEs) such as poverty, bereavement, and addiction. Attachment matters because it affects not only how safe we feel, our ability to regulate our emotions and stress, our adaptability, resilience, and lifelong mental and physical health, but attachment style can also be passed on. In addition, this paper utilizes attachment theory to speculate on the likely attachment styles for the three generations of the Parker family and looks at the possible parenting behavior in the first two, the effect of alcoholism and the intergenerational impact of trauma and depression.

Keywords: genealogy; family history; attachment; depression; trauma; prolonged grief disorder; adverse childhood experiences; alcoholic; alcohol use disorder; bereavement

1. Introduction

In 2013, I discovered that my grandfather Walter Parker's home in The Tank Yard, Thorney, Cambridgeshire, England, had become a museum. The day I visited, a volunteer steward told me about a cousin named Mary (born in 1918) who he thought would be delighted to meet me. Mary welcomed me as family and an important bridge to her past. Nearing the end of her life, she had lost most of her sight and was, as she said, "sliding toward death" in a "comfortable" nursing home. She had outlived her peers, husband, and only child, while her remaining sister had Alzheimer's disease. In the 1920s, Mary's uncle Walter taught her to ice skate, and as she told me about that winter, her face lit up. In her remaining years, Mary brought alive the "model" Victorian village of her childhood, built, and still owned by the Dukes of Bedford. As I absorbed the stories, I saw with delight that Mary found unexpected meaning and new purpose in relating the joys, domestic details, and tragedies woven into our family's daily life.

Later, I was not surprised to learn that sharing family history can boost one's mood and create bonds of common interest (Moore et al. 2020); but genealogy can do much more. According to Evans (2021, p. 101), "family history reconstructs memories about family lives in the past and in that process reveals the ... secret keeping, emotional familial management, and its impact on people in the past and present". I propose that any psychological insight genealogists uncover can give individuals new opportunities to thrive and pass on a healthier psychological legacy. Indeed, historian Emma Shaw reports in her article *Who we are and why we do it* that the goal of some family historians is "to uncover any inheritable ... traits and/or conditions that may impact negatively on those in the present. For these respondents, family history research was a tool in which certain medical traits could be identified, traced, and perhaps eradicated" (Shaw 2020, p. 119). In *How do Family Historians Work with Memory?*, public historian Tanya Evans quotes author Betty O'Neil, "family history is a microhistory, an individual and family experience of a particular time in history and geography that reflects many of the larger national, transactional and global themes" (Evans 2021, p. 98). For me, a motif around mental health, particularly depression, resonated most strongly. It first emerged from conversations with my cousin Mary, who described relatives who struggled with their psychological well-being and reminded me of the depressive episodes my mom and I suffered. I submit that family history knowledge can allow us to recognize and challenge maladaptive behavior, makes available important medical information, and opens the possibility to reverse a negative or toxic psychological inheritance and bring about positive change, whether self-directed or guided by mental health professionals, thereby allowing us to leave a more positive psychological legacy.

My mother, Doreen (born 1938), rationalized the distant relationship she had with her father in part due to his age of 51 when she was born. She also told me how Walter's social and emotional development had been interrupted by decades spent in an isolated homestead on the Canadian Prairies, leaving him firmly trapped in the Victorian mind-set of his youth. However, in this paper, I consider the lives of three generations: Ann, Walter, and Ann Parker through the lens of attachment theory and the impact his mother's poverty, bereavement, depression, and alcoholism had on him and his daughter, Doreen. This is important because attachment has lifelong consequences and attachment styles can be passed down the generations. I believe such investigations can help family historians bring toxic secrets and patterns of belief and behavior into the open, so that genealogists can weave them into their own narrative in the hope that this process lessens or brings to an end intergenerational trauma (Evans 2021, p. 100).

2. Results the Method Employed

The method employed was to collate births, deaths, causes of death, census records, reports from the Huntingdon Archive, interviews of people who knew Ann, Walter and Doreen and the author's own memories. The experience of each is related in the narrative and summarized in Table 1 below. I consider adverse childhood experience (ACE) studies that find links between the number of adversities and adult psychological health (including alcoholism) and physical health outcomes (Felitti 2002) as well as the impacts of traumatic loss, bereavement, depression, and alcoholism. I set these against the historical backdrop of migration, the Great Depression, and the Second World War by linking them to corroborating information—for example around living alone (Walter), being unusually self-reliant (Walter and teenage Doreen) and a brief description of Doreen's mother, Hilda. This paper utilizes attachment theory to speculate on likely attachment styles and parenting behavior.

Table 1. Summary of three generations of the Parker family.

Name; Birth; Occupation; Marriage; Death; Cause of Death	Places Lived	Proposed Attachment Style. Adverse Childhood Experiences (ACEs)[1] Loss/Trauma	Mental Health
First generation (4.1) **Name** Ann Parker née Bates **Birth** 1856 Alconbury-Cum-Weston, Huntingdonshire, England. **Occupation** Domestic servant. **Marriage** 1880 St Peter's, Upwell, Norfolk. **Death** 1938 Thorney, Cambridgeshire. **Cause of Death** Fibroid degeneration of the heart	Alconbury-Cum-Weston, Huntingdonshire, England. Upwell, Norfolk; Thorney, Cambridgeshire.	Avoidant attachment style. Childhood lived in poverty. Three siblings died before Ann's birth, (from meningitis, unknown cause, and fever). Age 2, brother Alfred died at 8 months; Tabes Mesenterica. Age 4, mother died; phthisis (consumption). Age 6 father remarries. Before age 7, sister Mary moves away. Age 7, sister Mary marries. 1873–1874, father and stepmother and 2 half siblings moved in and out of the workhouse. 1875, father dies in the workhouse. 1876, stepmother dies in workhouse. 1883, firstborn Lily Ann dies at 18 months old, TB meningitis.	Alcoholic; depression
Second generation (4.2) **Name** Walter Parker **Occupations** Agricultural laborer; apprenticeship carpenter and joiner; homesteader; joiner for the London, Midland and Scottish Railway, Sheffield; after retirement, worked for a garage until aged 89 years. **Birth** 1885, Upwell, Norfolk. **Marriage** 1936, St Mary's, Sheffield, now the cathedral. **Death** 1975, Arkley, Hertfordshire. **Cause of Death** Cardiac arrest; congested heart failure.	Upwell, Norfolk. Thorney, Cambridgeshire. Homestead Nw-22-24-7 West, Canada; Ashern, Manitoba, Canada. Edmund Road, Sheffield. Arkley, Barnet, Hertfordshire.	Dismissing-avoidant attachment style. 1883, death of sister before his birth. Alcoholic mother. 1909–1931, isolation on the Canadian Prairies. 1939–1945, heavy duty squad WW2. 1940, Sheffield Blitz.	Depression, lifelong smoker.
Third generation (4.3) **Name** Doreen Parker **Occupation** nurse **Birth** 1938, Sheffield. **Marriage** 1958, St Mary's, Sheffield, now the cathedral. **Death** 2002, Swindon, Wiltshire. **Cause of Death** Deep Vein Thrombosis; Ovarian Cancer.	Edmund Road, Sheffield. Nurses home, King Edward VII Orthopaedic Hospital, Rivelin. Nurses home, City General Hospital, Sheffield. High Storrs, Sheffield. Arkley, Barnet, Hertfordshire. Marlborough, Wiltshire.	Securely attached to mother Hilda. Avoidant attachment to Walter. Grew up in poverty with a Victorian father. 1939–1945, WW2. 1940, Sheffield Blitz. Bullied at grammar school. Left home at 16 and moved into nurse's home. Bullied during her later years of nurse training. 1962, miscarriage. 1969, closet friend emigrates. c1972, death of closest friend.	Depression, battled with excess weight. Smoker.

2.1. Attachment Theory

Attachment theory was first proposed in the 1950s by British psychoanalyst John Bowlby. According to Bowlby, infants discover how safe, available, and trustworthy people are during their early months and years. Given a child's "immense and profound need to survive, a child will always develop an attachment relationship with his or her caregiver(s), no matter what the caregiver's characteristics are" (Blair-Gómez 2013, p. 36). Mary Main explained that if the important people in an infant's life are insensitive, cold, rejecting, unpredictable, or frightening, the child learns that others "cannot be counted on for support and comfort, and this knowledge is embodied in insecure or anxious working models of attachment" (Main quoted in Fraley and Shaver 2000, p. 3). Main added that the insecure child could excessively demand attention and care or withdraw from others and attempt a high degree of self-sufficiency. In contrast, an infant who is cared for in an attuned and consistent way develops a secure attachment and can live their life expecting others will be available when needed (Feeney et al. 2008).

Attachment theory is important in understanding our ancestors because "although a secure attachment can be gained through positive relationships in later life, our original attachment style often stays with us over our lifetime and can be transmitted in some form or other to subsequent generations" (Parker-Drabble 2020). So, what kind of attachment did Walter have to his mother, Ann? Modern parents who struggle with unresolved loss can display "a range of perplexing behaviors during parenting, including dissociative-like stilling, distorted and frightening facial and vocal expressions, and poorly timed, rough, or intrusive caregiving" (Fearon 2004, p. 255). However, Griffin (2020) pointed out that historically "harsh and distant mothering was not regarded as problematic or abnormal" but was part of a "widely shared cultural belief within many working-class families that mothers should not overindulge their children." This confusion between meeting children's emotional needs and spoiling or indulging them continued. Indeed, "psychoanalytic and behaviorist theories of the 1940s and 1950s presumed that infants would be clingier and more dependent the more their needs were satisfied" (Duschinsky 2020), whereas Blatz's work demonstrated that when children are confident their needs will be met, they become increasingly independent (Duschinsky 2020).

Canadian psychologist Mary Ainsworth (1913–1999) developed the "strange situation" procedure in order to observe the variety of attachment styles exhibited between mothers and children (Ainsworth and Bell 1970; Seymour 2013). In the procedure, the behaviors of 100 infants aged between 12 and 18 months were observed using one-way glass in eight situations lasting three minutes each. Ainsworth discovered that approximately 60% of the children became upset when the mother left the room but when she returned, the child actively sought the parent and was easily comforted. Children who exhibit this pattern of behavior are labeled "secure" and tend to have parents who are responsive to their needs. Around 20% or less of infants appeared uncomfortable when the stranger was in the room; and when separated from their mother, they became extremely distressed. When these children were reunited with their parents, they were difficult to soothe, often exhibiting conflicting behaviors that suggested they wanted to be comforted and "punish" the parent for leaving. These children are often called anxious-resistant. The third pattern of attachment that Ainsworth et al. documented was referred to as avoidant. Avoidant children (about 20% of the group) did not appear particularly distressed by the separation. When the mother returned, these infants avoided seeking contact with their parents. Children who appear insecure (anxious-resistant or avoidant) often have parents who are either insensitive to their needs or inconsistent or rejecting in their caretaking style. Ballard (1993) found that children of alcoholic mothers were more likely to have an avoidant attachment style than children of non-alcoholic mothers.

According to Reisz et al. (2018), Bowlby later wrote about disorganized attachment that can replace a previous attachment when the child feels threatened in specific ways. He identified three circumstances when this might happen, first where there is a threat conflict, i.e., when someone previously associated with safety becomes associated with threat, for example when a caregiver is holding a child down to allow a medical procedure. Second, where there is safe haven ambiguity. Here, even if there are no cues for threat this too can change a child's normal way of reacting; for example, when the child is in a new situation that may appear to have no end. A third circumstance is known as activation without assuagement and is activated when a child has a long-time need for a safe caregiver, but they do not appear to sooth the child or help them name and regulate their feelings and emotions. For example, this might happen when a child is institutionalized in a workhouse or isolation hospital. Bowlby noted James Robertson's observation that when hospitalized children returned home in these circumstances, a child usually experienced dysregulated rage and/or despair.

The consequence of these three experiences could lead to future disorganization when the child, or adult, experiences similar triggers, or has similar expectations, fears, or hopes evoked by the original circumstance. Bowlby noted in his clinical practice that "events could be kept from conscious attention. He used the term selective exclusion to refer to the way in which attention divides the field of awareness into the relevant and irrelevant, imaginable, and feasible" (Reisz et al. 2018, p. 122). In the short term, this may protect our ancestors from overload and further disorganization. However, Bowlby saw this need for defensive exclusion as the root cause behind avoidance and if it is needed repeatedly, our relative may have lost important life information, affecting their emotional growth, their relationships, and the ability to keep themselves emotionally stable.

It can be difficult to picture our ancestors' parenting, but Ann's alcoholism gives us an additional clue because we know that alcoholics rarely have securely attached children. According to Vungkhanching et al. (2004), children of alcoholics are at increased risk for attachment difficulties. As most addicts manifest immense distrust in their relationships, often avoiding emotional openness and intimacy with others, it seems likely that Ann had a problematic relationship with her children.

2.2. Dysfunctional Family

To manage the stress of a dysfunctional home life, Wegscheider (1981) proposed five personality styles in children of alcoholics: Hero, Scapegoat, Lost Child, Mascot, and Enabler.[2] In this model, the Hero, often the eldest, takes responsibility and is usually a high achiever, a perfectionist, and/or a people pleaser. The Scapegoat is a rebellious and disruptive individual whose role is to take the spotlight away from the alcoholic parent. The Lost Child adapts by unknowingly repressing their thoughts, feelings, and needs, withdrawing into themselves, needing less adult attention, and often being overlooked. Lost Children may grow up to avoid intimate relationships, guard against anxiety or abandonment, and be fearful of risk or initiative. Perhaps Walter, who his nieces believed to be a shy, quiet lad, became the Lost Child, emotionally left to himself. The Mascot is the family clown who takes attention away from the dysfunction. They try to make people laugh despite the unaddressed psychological pain within the family. Finally, the role of Enabler makes all the other roles possible. They try to keep everyone happy, usually at the expense of their own needs. From my conversations with Mary, this role seems to have been fulfilled by Walter's father, Stephen. "He would do anything for anybody" and "tried to give his wife the best life he could."

An addict's family often develops unspoken rules such as "Don't talk, don't feel, don't trust." They commonly exhibit mood swings, along with inconsistent and erratic behavior. According to an article on the King University website, when drug or alcohol abuse exists in a family, "family rules, roles, and relationships are established and organized around the alcoholic and/or other substances, in an effort to maintain the family's homeostasis and balance."[3] Individual family members can believe they have become adept at managing the alcoholic's behavior and are protecting the "shameful" secret of dependence. Instead, the behavior can lead to a cycle of insecure attachment, a predisposition to addiction, and learnt, damaging co-dependent patterns of behavior that may become part of the next generation's inheritance.

3. Three Generations of the Parker Family

"Research shows that the adversity we experience as a child can affect how our stress response functions, leading to long-term changes in our brains and bodies and leading to health problems as an adult. Experiencing 4 or more [adverse childhood experiences] ACEs are associated with significantly increased risk for 7 out of 10 leading adult causes of death, including heart disease, stroke, cancer, COPD, diabetes, Alzheimer's disease and suicide."[4] Research carried out by Felitti (2002) linked drug addiction, hepatitis, fractures, obesity, and alcoholism to adverse childhood experiences. As a family historian exploring my ancestors' lives, I expect to learn something from the past that helps me in the present (see Table of three generations of the Parker family). I seek historical empathy that requires "one to imagine the other's situation and what it might feel like, while simultaneously recognizing one's difference from them" (Landsberg 2009, p. 223). This differs from projecting our own beliefs, thoughts, and experiences on to our ancestors. It is more the "ability to appreciate the other person's feelings without yourself becoming so emotionally involved that your judgment is affected" (Lanzoni 2015). Its value is in creating what Alison Landsberg describes as prosthetic memory, one that is created from others' memories acquired from not only personal accounts, but also through mass culture. Through these means, we can understand past attitudes and ambitions, and the resultant empathy can become a tool for contemporary understanding (Craddock et al. 2018, p. 16).

3.1. Ann Catherine Parker (1856–1938)

Ann grew up in poverty and her young life was threaded with tragedy, but family historians know her experience was far from unique. However, research by Felitti et al. (2019) tells us that the number of adverse childhood experiences (ACEs) one has affects how we each respond to stress. This leads to long-term changes in the brain and body and to subsequent health problems as an adult. As we read about our ancestors' lives, it is worth noting that an adverse childhood experience includes the loss or separation of a parent or sibling, poverty, accident, or invasive medical treatment. We should also bear in mind that experiencing four or more ACEs is associated with significantly increased risk for 7 out of 10 leading adult causes of death, including heart disease, stroke, cancer, chronic obstructive pulmonary disease, diabetes, Alzheimer's disease and suicide. Earlier, Felitti (2002) specifically linked drug addiction, hepatitis, fractures, obesity, and alcoholism to adverse childhood experiences.

When she was four years old, Ann's mother died of consumption. Although we cannot know Ann's relationship with her mother, we know consumption kills slowly, so we can hypothesize that the attachment break when death came was traumatic. It would therefore have been natural for Ann to be anxious about the mortality of close family members. Saphire-Bernstein et al. have linked an inheritable gene to optimism, self-esteem, and mastery: the belief that one has control over one's own life. They further note that these three psychological resources "have been found to be significant predictors of effective stress management, neurophysiological responses to stress, and physical and psychological health-related outcomes" (Saphire-Bernstein et al. 2011, p. 15120). According to them, optimism, self-esteem, and mastery are critical psychological resources for coping well with stress and depression. However, McEwen and Akil (2020) reminds us that while it is not possible to "erase the biological consequences of experience, an individual's trajectory can be modified by additional experiences that can either enhance their ability to cope in a healthy manner or lead them to succumb to stress-related disorders" (McEwen and Akil 2020, p. 15). Sadly, Ann was unable to avoid alcoholism or cardiovascular disease.

Bowlby recognized that in grief and loss, a child uses their attachment style to cope with adversity and regain their sense of security. But who could Ann have turned to after the death of her mother? The 1861 Census shows Ann's then-only sister, Mary, was living with her in the family home. It is probable Mary was a mother figure for Ann, but Mary must have had her own issues. She, too, had experienced a multitude of adverse childhood experiences. Three of Mary's younger siblings had died before Ann's birth and at six years old Mary was listed as present at her five-year-old brother's death. It cannot have been easy for Mary to look after the impoverished family before and after her mother's death.

By the time Ann reached the age of six, her father had remarried. This relationship would have been particularly important because by the time Ann was seven, her sister Mary, aged 20, was married and living 30 miles away. Sotero (2006) and Colich et al. (2020) discovered that the physiological and psychological effects of overwhelming emotional experiences affect a person's lifelong health (Sotero 2006, p. 99).[5] It is therefore likely that Ann's development, resilience, and long-term well-being were threatened by the death of her mother and siblings as well as her sister's move. Did Ann's ability to form close emotional attachments diminish after each loss? Ann's granddaughter, Mary, told me she could not recall a single time when Ann had laughed or even smiled, which reminded me of the first ever episode of Who Do You Think You Are? in 2004.[6] The program described conservationist Bill Oddie's mother as an undemonstrative, difficult woman. Like Ann Parker she had suffered the loss of an infant. Mary remembered Ann as an unhappy alcoholic who was volatile and "difficult to get along with."[7] Mary shared Bill Oddie's sentiment, "I wish I knew then what I know now, because I could have made a difference". Tragically, in Mary's case she had not been able to help her only child survive depression.

In England, school was not free or compulsory, and in Ann's poverty-stricken family she would have started work as soon as it could be found. The Census record of 1871 shows 15-year-old Ann had left Alconbury Weston, Huntingdon, and followed her sister to Upwell in Norfolk. Ann worked as a servant for a 63-year-old farmer and reported to the live-in housekeeper. Ann's move did not save her from further loss. Both her father and stepmother died in the workhouse before Ann's marriage to Stephen Parker in 1880. In October 1883, Stephen and Ann's firstborn died of tubercular meningitis at 18 months, when Ann was approximately 24 weeks pregnant with her second child, Ethel.

In light of her sister Mary's loss of four babies, it is plausible that Ann may have viewed the birth of her children with some ambivalence and distress, which could have been transmitted to Walter (Yehuda and Lehrner 2018). Certainly, it seems that Ann paid an emotional price for the traumas she suffered. Although there is a common belief that our ancestors were less affected by loss, disaster, and trauma than we are, Hilary Marland, professor of history at the Center for the History of Medicine at the University of Warwick, makes a convincing case that poverty contributed to and exacerbated the mental suffering of women in Victorian Britain (Strange 2006, p. 471). That the poor were somehow immune to the loss of their loved ones is also soundly contested by Julie-Marie Strange, professor of modern British history at Durham University. In her book about death, grief, and poverty, Strange (2012) explained that poverty increased rather than deadened the anguish of the poor.

While it is possible Ann resolved her trauma and integrated a new understanding that allowed her to respond differently to her children, it is more likely that the traumas associated with her loses weakened her resilience to what was to come. It is impossible to say if Ann's parenting was considered unusual toward the end of the nineteenth century, but genealogists would probably understand if Ann unconsciously emotionally distanced herself from Walter and his siblings to protect herself from further loss.

3.1.1. Ann's Addiction to Alcohol

Although Ann's grandchildren, Mary, and Rene believed she was addicted to alcohol all her adult life, neither knew the trigger.[8] Ann's alcohol use disorder was not named within the family but referred to as Ann's "condition." Vaillant (2009) suggested a challenging childhood environment "is an important predictor of when an individual loses control of alcohol." Nickerson et al. (2013) noted that "the younger the child was at the time of loss [of a parent], the more likely the child was to develop mental health problems, including anxiety, mood, or substance abuse issues" (see also Lovett 2014). Therefore, Ann's bereavements or fear for her children's lives may have made her more vulnerable to alcohol misuse disorder and poor mental health.[9] The Austrian neurologist and founder of psychoanalysis, Sigmund Freud, described "melancholia as an acutely painful and unresolved form of mourning, associated with 'self-reproaches', 'self revilings'[sic], and 'a delusional expectation of punishment'" (quoted in Lapping 2019). In a more recent study, Solomon (2001) has explained that the same genes and neural pathways that can make us more vulnerable to depression are also involved in anxiety, alcoholism, and suicide.[10]

Why did Ann drink to excess? Schindler (2019) showed that alcohol might be used to reduce social fears and help those with a preoccupied style of attachment feel closer to others. Individuals with preoccupied (sometimes called ambivalent/enmeshed/anxious) attachments often try to elicit care and support through clinging and controlling behavior (Shaver and Hazan 1993). These efforts at closeness are not only used to establish physical contact but aim to foster a sense of intimacy, similarity, and oneness with a romantic partner (Mikulincer and Shaver 2003). Such strategies are also indicated by an overdependence on relationship partners (Shaver and Hazan 1993) and the preoccupied person's belief that they are helpless and incompetent at managing their own feelings (Mikulincer and Florian 1998). These individuals can also be preoccupied with their own distress and other people's availability to help them cope. "Avoidant or fearful individuals, on the other hand, are uncomfortable with closeness and might use higher doses [of alcohol] to avoid contact and deactivate emotions" (Schindler 2019, p. 727). People with an avoidant style lack attachment security and are compulsively self-reliant, with a preference for staying emotionally distant from others. Reisz et al. (2018) pointed out that "avoidance is a rigid, brittle form of organization with significant disadvantages, such as not seeking help when needed or even registering the need for help."

However, while a child's relationship with their parents is considered important, other factors should be considered. The research of Fraley and Shaver (1997) on adult attachment revealed two avoidant groups. The first group, fearfully avoidant, are afraid of emotional bonds and feel high anxiety, but can long to be in a loving relationship. The second group is known as dismissing avoidant. According to Connors (1997), dismissing avoidants believe "renunciation of love is preferable to the pain and [perceived] danger of relationship; instead, they seek control and mastery over the environment" (Connors 1997, p. 476). Dismissing avoidant adults experience low anxiety and do not fear rejection or loneliness. Indeed, Fraley and Shaver discovered that when dismissing individuals were instructed to suppress their thoughts and feelings; they were able to minimize the attention they paid to thoughts. After speaking to two of Ann's grandchildren—Mary and Rene—at length, I wondered if Ann had an avoidant style. Walter appears to fit the description of the dismissing avoidant style.

Although Ann's demeanor as described by Mary and Rene cannot be symptomatic of an alcohol use disorder, we can surmise that the emotional blows Ann received, and a likely insecure attachment style, diminished Ann's ability to cope with the tragic death of her first child. Given that children currently brought up in poverty are at an equal risk of forming an insecure or disorganized attachment as children who have been mistreated (Voges et al. 2019), it would appear unlikely that Ann grew up with secure attachments. It would have been remarkable if Ann had avoided anxiety or depression, either or both of which could have been the precursor to her drinking, possibly triggered by postnatal depression or genetic inheritance (Prescott et al. 2000, p. 808; Womersley et al. 2021, pp. 33–34).[11]

3.1.2. Grief

It is also possible that Ann suffered from a prolonged grief disorder (PGD). Researchers have explored how symptoms of PGD and depression co-occur in the bereaved. Kokou-Kpolou et al. (2021) have looked at the this in light of the revised definition of PGD in the new edition of Diagnostic and Statistical Manual of Mental Disorders (*DSM–5*) (Boelen et al. 2020, p. 1771008). Kokou-Kpolou's investigations might be particularly useful because it is a nonwestern study in a "region of the world where the mortality rate is very high and consequently bereavement issues are a major health concern" (Kokou-Kpolou et al. 2021). The researchers also considered the potential impact of sociocultural and religious factors. Their findings might therefore raise possibilities about Ann's possible experience. Their results "identified a resilient class (20.6%), predominantly PGD class (44.7%), and combined PGD/Depression class (34.7%) . . . age, time elapsed since the loss, continuing bond and relationship with the deceased, as well as spirituality were the differential predictors of class membership" (Kokou-Kpolou et al. 2021) "Younger people were found to be more at-risk to endorse pervasive symptomatology." More recently, bereaved individuals were likely to belong to the PGD class, and those who mourned the death of an immediate family member were more likely to belong to the combined

PGD/Depression class. Those in these later classes also reported a higher level of continuing bond with the deceased. Reading this, I was reminded that the large elaborate funeral card given to Ann and Stephen in 1883 after the death of their daughter is the only item associated with Ann that has survived. Could this be indicative of an association between bereavement complications and high levels of post-loss attachment to the deceased found in the studies of Boulware and Bui (2016) and Gillies and Neimeyer (2006)? Lower levels of spiritual beliefs were associated with the predominantly PGD class, which might be associated with a difficulty in accepting and finding meaning in the loss. Kokou-Kpolou pointed out that a belief in a god or understanding death to be an integral part of human existence "may offer comfort and consolation at time of loss and facilitate the mourning process" (Kokou-Kpolou et al. 2021).

Others have looked at the impact of grief and attachment style. According to Maccallum and Bryant (2018), "it is possible that attachment avoidance contributes to bereavement complications, such as depression, by reducing the likelihood that an individual will utilize available social supports or develop new attachments." Furthermore, Lai et al. (2015) found that "female gender, high levels of depression, and preoccupation with relationships significantly predicted higher levels of prolonged grief risk." Sochos and Aleem went further in their finding that where there is complicated grief parental attachment insecurity may facilitate that transmission intergenerationally (Sochos and Aleem 2021, p. 14).

3.2. Walter Parker (1885–1975)
3.2.1. Possible Consequences of Ann's Trauma

We know that the effects of a parent's unresolved trauma can be passed on to their children. Author Marianne Hirsch described 'postmemory' as "the relationship of the second generation to powerful, often traumatic, experiences that preceded their births but that were nevertheless transmitted to them so deeply as to seem to constitute memories in their own right" (Hirsch 2008, p. 103). While I have no evidence of this for Walter, given the ongoing danger of meningitis, TB, fever, and more, which led to Ann's losses, it seems almost inevitable that Walter too was aware that he or his sisters, cousins, and peers could also die young.[12] According to Beiner (2014), intensive "remembrance is retained beyond personal recollections of those who experienced historical events and can be transmitted over three generations as a fluid 'communicative memory' (in which grandparents pass on vivid narratives to grandchildren and their peers) before it is formulated into a more stable form" (Beiner 2014, p. 303). Although an awareness of death is likely to be intermittent, it was not only family, friends, and neighbors who could bring it to the forefront.[13] Newspapers also reminded people of their mortality through the annual death report in each area as well as the daily obituaries report.[14]

Traumatized parents can struggle with debilitating depression, unexplained grief, and an increased vulnerability to stress without understanding the cause (Kirmayer et al. 2000). It was sobering to learn that "the absence of emotional support early in a mother's life, years before conception, are also associated with neural changes . . . in her offspring shortly after birth" (Hendrix et al. 2021, p. 470) "found that the more emotional neglect a mother had experienced during her own childhood, the more strongly her baby's amygdala was connected to the frontal cortical regions" "which has been associated with an increased risk for depression and anxiety across the lifespan" (Elsevier 2021; Hendrix et al. 2021, p. 470). Therefore, it is reasonable to consider that Walter and his siblings may have inherited intergenerational consequences from their mother's early life adversity and depending on their life experiences, passed a toxic legacy onto their children.

Another consequence of Ann's experiences could have been an inability to react appropriately to her children.

Iyengar et al. comments:

"A mother with preoccupied unresolved trauma may be hyper-vigilant in response to her infant's distress, while a mother with a denied unresolved trauma may under-respond to her infant's distress". (Iyengar et al. 2019, p. 110)

Kim et al. (2014) also studied mothers with unresolved trauma, discovering that the amygdala, the part of the brain that processes emotion and memory, was turned on when viewing unknown children but was turned off when the mother looked at her child's distressed or happy face. We can speculate that this inability to recognize her children's suffering protected Ann from reexperiencing her own trauma but could have left Walter and his sisters psychologically "alone," with no mother to mitigate or help process their emotional pain (Iyengar et al. 2019, p. 110). This unconscious defense mechanism could also explain, in part, how a transgenerational transmission of trauma can be inherited.

According to Sochos and Aleem (2021), "both parental attachment anxiety and avoidance increase the impact of parental complicated grief on child traumatic stress." Anxiously attached parents who also struggle themselves to accept an important loss would be expected to display more exaggerated parental inconsistency between overprotecting and emotionally neglecting the child. On the other hand, avoidant parents tend to suppress negative emotion both in themselves and their children (Edelstein and Shaver 2004) and would be expected to do so more intensely when they also experience sadness and despair relating to an unresolved loss." (Sochos and Aleem 2021, p. 14). We can also consider that Sochos and Aleem concluded "Psychological vulnerability in bereaved young persons was associated with an insecure parental attachment style (Sochos and Aleem 2021, p. 15)."

3.2.2. Walter's Attachment Style

Bowlby postulated that people with attachment-related avoidance—those who withdraw from a parent—prefer not to rely on other people or open up to others when they are distressed. Considering the work of Bowlby and Ainsworth, we might conclude, as well as we can, that Walter had a dismissing avoidant attachment style, perhaps echoing his mother's style (Kelley et al. 2010, p. 1558). Certainly, Zelekha and Yaakobi (2020) found that the more avoidant the mother, the greater likelihood the male in the next generation will be avoidant. Kelley et al. discovered that people who suspected their mothers of alcoholism reported a more avoidant overall attachment style in romantic relationships (Kelley et al. 2010, p. 1565). However, we should not assume Walter did not need to feel close to people, rather that he had buried his need (Carvallo and Gabriel 2020). Perhaps because Walter did not appear to suffer from painful rumination, he could be perceived by others as uncaring (Turan et al. 2016, p. 234).

As avoidant parents tend to distance themselves emotionally from distressing events and experiences, their bereaved children may also adopt that strategy (Grossmann 1989). However, emotionally distant, avoidant parents provide relatively consistent care, potentially helping their children maintain a sense of stability as they deal with the disruption of death (Sochos and Aleem 2021, p. 13).

3.2.3. Ann's Alcoholism and Depression

Nineteenth-century opinions of alcoholism were replete with moralistic overtones. Professor of modern British history, Emma Griffin notes in her book *Bread Winner* that "drinking was quite easily incorporated into narratives about fathers, but alcoholic mothers were an object of shame" (Griffin 2020, p. 248). In 1878, Ann may have been aware of the feeling a female writer expressed when she wrote that a man should be excused of domestic abuse if he had the "universally condemned creature, the drunken wife" (Cobbe 1878, p. 69). One can imagine the humiliation and shame Walter and his siblings might have felt at having an alcoholic mother. Walter was likely deeply affected by Ann's understandable depression. A paper from Lupien et al. explained that depressed mothers "have been associated with reductions in overall sensitivity to the infant, and with an increased rate of withdrawn, disengaged behaviors" (Lupien et al. 2011, p. 14324). A child of a depressed mother can be so adversely affected that their enlarged amygdala is comparable to the changes found in an infant's brain when a mother has been wholly absent from their life. Qin et al. (2014) reports that high childhood anxiety is associated with enlarged amygdala volume. Further, "sustained anxiety in children may bias this system toward withdrawal or avoidance behavior to alleviate anxious states."

3.2.4. Mitigating Factors

Whatever happened in Walter's childhood, ground-breaking research by Zelekha and Yaakobi (2020) suggests optimistic possibilities. These researchers provided empirical evidence that stable experiences throughout adulthood—for example, the birth of a child or changes in income and employment status—are likely to moderate intergenerational transmission and influence people's attachment orientation in adulthood. Zelekha's team explored the positive role that "intimates, friends, and even the work environment" can have in changing attachment style, making attachment a lifelong process rather than a condition fixed in childhood (Zelekha and Yaakobi 2020, p. e0233906).

Furthermore, although Beletsis and Brown (1981) noted that female alcoholism is generally associated with personal problems and that higher numbers of depression and anxiety disorders are found in alcoholic women (quoted in Saatcioglu et al. 2006), Qin et al. discovered:

> ... changes may confer some adaptive advantages for developing balanced strategies to cope with challenging and stressful situations in real life. (Qin et al. 2014, p. 898)

It is clear that Walter's young life was not solely dysfunctional. His parents, teachers, community, and early employers helped him gain practical skills. Indeed, Simpson and Belsky (2008) suggested that the "inborn attachment bias can be channeled in different directions and can [also] be either secure or insecure as a function of the way parents prepare [their offspring] to survive and adapt to a specific bio-ecological niche" (Zelekha and Yaakobi 2020, p. e0233906). The consistent nurturing, acceptance, and encouragement that Walter's granddaughters described receiving from their grandfather may have mitigated the negative effects of Ann's behavior in Walter. This desire on my part is not without basis in scholarship, as attachment theory allows that children can have different attachment styles with each caregiver, and Zelekha and Yaakobi (2020) commented that fathers and mothers have differing effects on their male and female attachment orientations. Strange reported that shared experiences between fathers and sons helped them to (re)discover a common language when they took up apprenticeships or joined the world of work (Strange 2012, p. 1020). Walter's agricultural work and his apprenticeships echoed his father's successful path in providing for a wife and family, which may have created an additional bond between them.

We know that Stephen moved away from his home village, where he appeared to have a good living as a carpenter and builder. It is important to consider that Stephen's duties for the Duke of Bedford in Thorney might have allowed him a closer relationship with his children, because he probably worked more predictable and fewer hours than he had when he was self-employed and likely ate all his meals with his family.

3.2.5. Walter Comes of Age

In 1907, at the age of 21, Walter left The Tank Yard in the close-knit Thorney village for Canada. He likely wore a money belt under a full set of thermal underwear and carried a rucksack on his back that was packed with a new leather notebook, a multi-purpose pen knife, a fork, a tin mug and plate, a flask of water, a cutthroat razor, brush and soap, a flannel, a change of clothes, and a set of basic carpentry tools. His companion was his neighbor and chum Ernie Kitchen, a recently qualified plumber. The two friends took out adjoining 160 acre plots and helped each other meet the stringent requirements to keep their land, but successful bachelor homesteaders were rare.[15] The men each had to cultivate at least 40 acres and build a permanent dwelling within three years of taking on their plot. This demand was brutal on the body, and the isolation and loneliness could cause great distress in even the hardiest pioneers (Joinson 2018). Homesteaders on the prairies of America and Canada were known to be at risk of prairie madness. In 1893, E.V. Smalley, the editor of Northwest Illustrated Monthly Magazine, said, "An alarming amount of insanity occurs in the new prairie States among farmers and their wives" (Joinson 2018) Walter's neighbor Ernie later traveled to England and returned with a wife, but reticent Walter kept a dog for company. Was Walter particularly at risk of prairie madness, given his inheritance from his depressed mother?

We know avoidant-attached adults tend to seek isolation and independence. But even without the isolation he experienced on the prairies, if Walter had an avoidant insecure attachment to his mother, he may have found it difficult to provide emotional support to others. Certainly, such adults can avoid relationships in an attempt to prevent disappointment and rejection. Was it also hard for him to trust and depend on people? Might Walter have unconsciously been escaping the discomfort of intimacy by creating a bachelor homestead on the prairie?

3.2.6. Walter's Return

Walter returned to England during the Great Depression. Jarrett (2019) pointed out that "mid-life—when anxiety and avoidance tend to decline—is arguably the time when we are most invested in various social roles and relationships". True or not, 51-year-old Walter was to propose marriage to a 36-year-old spinster housekeeper. According to my mother, Hilda asked newly arrived Walter to help her when she tragically found her employer hanging in an out-building. Their relationship blossomed despite its macabre beginning, and they kept in touch, although Hilda had to move to take up a live-in job in Welwyn Garden City, England, while Walter found them a home.

In the 1930s, those without qualifications, skills, or family to rely on lived in a desperate state. For a time, Walter moved in with his elderly parents, who supported themselves with a small parlor shop that sold single cigarettes, tobacco, and sweets in twists of paper. Walter struggled to find long-term work and clung to his hard-won savings, not knowing how long it would be before he found secure employment. Understanding how difficult it would be to find affordable board and lodgings, he concentrated his search in an area where he had family. Before his marriage to Hilda, Walter's training and experience as a carpenter and joiner enabled him to secure work for the London, Midland, and Scottish Railway. He lodged with his youngest sister Lucy, brother-in-law Fred Snr (a war hero), and nephew Fred Jnr. I expect his bed was in the attic space of the two up, two down terrace half a mile from the Sheffield Midland station in the center of industrial Sheffield. It is difficult to imagine a starker contrast with village life in Thorney or his life in Canada.

Another desperate act touched Walter and Hilda's life when his brother-in-law lay down in front of a steam engine. The family story is that Fred Snr could not live with the shame of his infidelity. The coroner ruled his death an accident, despite indications that it was not. which allowed insurance to pay for the funeral. However, Lucy could not support herself and her son in Sheffield, so they returned to Ann and Stephen in Thorney. Walter took over the tenancy agreement of Lucy's small, terraced house with an outdoor privy.[16] He now had a secure job and a home and could marry Hilda.

Earlier, I concluded that Walter might have had a dismissing avoidant attachment style that an attentive father could have somewhat mitigated. During the decades Walter spent mostly alone in Canada, his style was unlikely to have changed. Whatever Walter's attachment style, I surmise from his bachelor homesteading in Manitoba that he was mostly self-sustaining and comfortable, without a physically present relationship. On his return to England, I imagine Walter made a pragmatic decision and looked for a spouse who would manage their domestic arrangements with whatever housekeeping money he gave her. This would not have been too out of step. In the early 1930s, The Matrimonial Post and Fashionable Marriage Advertiser established in 1860 still showed how important gendered roles were in hopeful readers. A "commitment to domesticity was paramount: both spinsters and bachelor clients requested "homely" individuals" and "steadiness was a much sought-after attribute." Walter may also have expected a younger wife to care for him in his old age. Women of the period looked for "a husband capable of providing reliable financial support and a home within which to bring up a family" (Langhamer 2013, pp. 24–25, 54). What marriage meant for Hilda is impossible to say, but it is worth noting that she was born when her father (another railway employee) was also 51 years of age and the age difference between her mother and father was very similar to the years between herself and Walter. Any sense of security Hilda's parents gave her was a memory, as both had died before she was 17 years old. Hilda spent much of her life living with an untreated thyroid condition, so swapping her role as a live-in housekeeper in a four-bedroom dwelling to become a wife living in a small terrace might have offered her much-appreciated security.[17] Cousin Mary said that Hilda had always wanted children but had given up hope of motherhood. Her successful pregnancy was remarkable, given she had hypothyroidism. I hope Hilda received more comfort and support from her husband than an avoidant attachment style might suggest.

3.3. Walter's Daughter Doreen Parker (1938–2002)
3.3.1. Doreen's Parents

Mom told me she was a welcome surprise for her 37-year-old mother but a shock to her father.[18] I do not know if Walter was reminded of his own childhood and whether this raised any demons from his past or fears that he thrust aside. In the last years of her life mom told me that she experienced Walter as "distant" and "emotionally absent." I expect Walter displayed some of his mother's parenting. Avoidantly attached individuals can feel burdened when asked to care for others, including their own children. This means they can be somewhat negligent, emotionally distant, and less responsive to their children, particularly if the children become highly distressed (Fraga 2018). When their offspring is most upset and in need of parental support, the avoidant parent may not have the skills to soothe and reassure their child. Doreen tried to get closer to her father, who as a son of an alcoholic, may have struggled to identify or convey his conscious feelings or the emotions he experienced. It would appear Walter could not be the father Mary believed her grandfather had been.

From about seven to nine months, infants will frequently have a special preference for a single attachment figure. The baby looks to this person for security, comfort, and protection.[19] No doubt Hilda was mom's primary attachment, but I believe Hilda also a had a tale to tell. Hilda had several live-in domestic jobs before her marriage. She presumably found a way to fit in, but two photos we have of her, one as a large, awkward teenager dwarfing her parents and the other in the uniform of a domestic servant trying to disappear into a hedge, suggest a young person who did not want to be seen. My impression is of a woman who was not sure of herself, and I was not surprised Mom told me that Hilda smothered her.

Meanwhile, I believe Walter's focus was to support his family in uncertain times, so he concentrated on his role as breadwinner. Although the workhouse system had come to an end in 1930, the newly named Public Assistance Institutions operated in a similar way. People continued to refer to the buildings as workhouses, and the dread of these cast a long-lasting shadow. With no work experience in England, no insurance, and a deep economic depression, my grandfather knew losing his job would cause his family severe hardship. The men who could not support their families had to surrender to the intrusion of comprehensive means testing carried out by insensitive officials in return for very little money. Walter saw this option as abhorrent charity and did everything he could to avoid receiving unemployment assistance.

3.3.2. Life in Sheffield

While Walter understood he had to live where there was work, he could not have felt a house in the industrial center of Sheffield, where gang wars had resulted in police brutality and corruption, was the best place to raise his child. Nor could he have seen much of Doreen, for he probably worked 48.6 h a week over six days, with overtime when he could get it (Huberman and Minns 2007, p. 542). When war broke out in September 1939, mothers with children under five were evacuated from cities and towns thought to be military targets. Those who had family they could stay with made their own arrangements.[20] Hilda told Doreen that they had evacuated for a short time.[21] As East Anglia had been proposed to accommodate refugees from Sheffield in 1938, Hilda might have thought it reasonable to take Doreen to her sister Minnie, living in the relative safety of Peterborough. However, it would have been a tight squeeze in the Matthews' little Victorian terrace, which already housed three adults and two children.

In 1921, the Canadian Census defined Walter as "Canadian", and it must have been hard for Walter to let this identity go. According to Rollero and Piccoli (2010, p. 199), it takes time for us to become a member of a new social group and to modify our identity, but in a few short years Walter had found work in a Depression, taken on a tenancy, married, learned to accommodate a wife and city living, become a father, and joined the heavy rescue squad. These experiences, Walter's age, and the danger to his family may have helped him reinvent himself and bond more easily with others. His work in the rescue squad was to shore up damaged walls and floors so the search for survivors could begin. Whatever Walter's attachment style in the few hours he was at home with his family, he would have been exhausted and it could have been difficult for him to be emotionally present.

Writing this article reminds me of the proverb, "It takes a village to raise a child." (Seymour 2013, p. 115). Research has shown the value of children having multiple attachments, but it takes different forms, according to the local environment and culture (Seymour 2013). While Walter may have found a sense of belonging through his work, Hilda and Doreen lived a much more restricted life at home. However, despite their austere life, I hope they found a welcoming community and friends at a local mother and baby clinic or in the shelters during a bombing raid (McIntosh 1997).

Walter and Hilda's psychological legacy and the poverty they endured meant their daughter was initially socially isolated, but her voracious reading was fueled by the weekly trip to the library with her parents. Doreen's knowledge grew and fed into the homework she poured over at the kitchen table. The Girl Guide movement offered her an escape from her claustrophobic home life, first as a Brownie and later as a Girl Guide. The movement aimed to encourage the development of the whole person. Doreen promised to 'help other people at all times' and obey the Guide Law which included vows to be trusted, loyal, thrifty, and to smile no matter what difficulties beset her.[22] She thrived in its no-nonsense practical environment. Doreen passed the competitive examination known as the eleven-plus, which gave her access to the local grammar school. Unlike some of her friends, she was able to take up her place because Walter paid for the expensive but compulsory school uniform. Although Walter was silent on the subject, I hope he knew that this support gave Doreen the chance to reinvent herself and apply for nurse training.

3.3.3. Doreen's Attachment Style

Conversations with my mom, Doreen, dad, and Doreen's lifelong friend, Sheila, led me to believe Hilda probably had an anxious or preoccupied attachment style to her mother, which gave her an "emotional hunger that unintentionally drained" Doreen and acted "as an unfulfilling substitute for real love and nurturance" for Hilda (Firestone 2013). Doreen experienced this as clinginess and a desire to be over-involved in her life, although Doreen welcomed the mothering she had from a friend's mother.[23] Hilda, desperate to hold onto her relationship with her daughter, sadly alienated her further by repeated, comprehensive apologies that encouraged Doreen to become fiercely independent.[24]

However, it is difficult to reach a conclusion about Doreen's attachment to Walter. I wonder if she had an avoidant attachment to Walter, as this has much to do with the emotional availability of a parent. Although her father did not physically neglect her, I suspect he avoided displays of emotion and intimacy and was mistuned to her emotional needs. Those with an avoidant attachment to a parent are often reserved and seem to back off when their child reaches out for support, affection, and reassurance. Walter probably felt overwhelmed and became increasingly distant when someone around him expressed strong feelings. Young Doreen might have expressed a need for closeness, but instead of receiving it, Walter withdrew. To a child, this can feel like a door has violently slammed in their face. Parents like Walter might not only avoid expressing their feelings, but they can also shut down their children's emotions by silent disapproval or lectures about how they need to grow up or toughen up. Given Walter's psychological inheritance, he might have particularly reacted to Doreen showing anxiety, fear, or sadness; instead, he might have expected her to be self-reliant, serious, and reserved. Doreen could have adapted by "developing a pseudo-independent stance (i.e., I can take care of myself)" (Firestone 2013).

The picture of Doreen's attachment to her father is confused, perhaps in part because Doreen left home at the age of 16 to train as an orthopedic nurse. Because she could not afford the bus fare home, Doreen experienced isolation at the hospital where she lived and worked. Children and adult patients with tuberculosis, congenital deformities, and poliomyelitis lived in the hospital for months, sometimes years. The attachments these children had to their family was broken, as the nursing profession, ignorant of children's attachment needs, gave the distraught children only the physical care they needed believing "within a few hours or a few days he would "settle down" [and] would "forget" his mother" (Barnett and Robertson 1991, p. 12). As children have a biological need to attach, it is understandable that they reached out to the young homesick nurses. Although professional distance was demanded from the students, they often eased their own loneliness and fulfilled their patients' need for meaningful connections in the quiet of the night shifts while they were in charge of the wards. The student nurses were taught to be observant of any change in their patient's condition. They were rigorous in their hygiene practices and were encouraged to predict what a patient needed before the patient knew they needed it. During the isolated and demanding training, Doreen became close to two nurses, and the small group became her surrogate family. Although the student nurses were ruled with a "rod of iron," their support of each other also led to games and singing and joking with patients.[25]

Doreen was a deeply empathic woman whose training gave her the tools to recognize people's needs and enable them, not just to cope but to thrive, despite their challenges. Mohammadreza Khodabakhsh explains, "empathy plays a key role in the nurse-patient relationship because it promotes an understanding of the patient's emotional status and perception and helps the nurse to effectively share or participate in the patient's experience" (Khodabakhsh 2012, p. 2). This ability to be empathic suggests Doreen's infant attachment with her mother was a secure one. Further evidence of a secure attachment may be Doreen's decision to deliberately choose roles where she had the most interaction with patients, rather than follow a career path that became managerial (Khodabakhsh 2012).

Nursing can attract compulsive adult caregivers who were defensive precocious caregivers in childhood (Taggart and Elsey 2021). But while Bowlby identified compulsive caregivers who deny their own needs and focus on the needs of others this does not fit my experience of Doreen (West and Keller 1991). She did not seek out or continually care for, or rescue others around her. Nor did Doreen appear to feel responsible for her parents. After leaving the family home aged 16 Doreen did not spend significant time with either parent until Walter moved into our family home when Doreen was 36 years old.

Although Doreen battled depression, I do not believe she knew of her grandmother Ann's trauma, catastrophic losses, alcoholism, or depression. If she had, I believe she would have recognized the intergenerational threads of anxiety and depression she and some of her cousins suffered. Neither Walter nor Doreen knew they had received a toxic psychological inheritance, but they both strived to give their children better parenting than they had known. Throughout Doreen's life, she was valued as a trusted, loyal, and thrifty person, and a safe attachment figure for some of the insecure adults around her who needed support. Mom often smiled no matter what anxiety, fear or difficulties beset her.

4. Conclusions

In this article, I explored three generations of the Parker family using key theories to show how a psychologically informed understanding of our ancestors can help family historians better understand their forebears, themselves, and living family. At the end of this research, I have come to believe each generation did what they could to leave a healthier legacy than the one they had inherited. Despite a difficult relationship with his mother, Walter grasped the opportunities his apprenticeship gave him. He emigrated and used his skill to build enough capital to become a farmer on the Canadian Prairie. Back in England, he did not expect to become a father, but he was able to support himself and his family during the Great Depression. However, Doreen grew up knowing her parents had few resources and that Walter and Hilda's future was precarious. I could not witness my grandfather Walter's informative years. Still, I wonder if what his daughter saw as Walter being an anachronism, an emotionally absent father stuck in the Victorian age, was as much about his psychological inheritance, attachment style, and the coping mechanisms he developed as a child.[26]

We cannot know our ancestors' psychological inheritance, that is the inherited traits, reactions, and patterns of behavior we inherit from our parents that are central to this paper. However, by the cautious exploration of theories, we can ask new questions and consider repeated patterns such as loss, depression, or addiction. With this information we can speculate about our ancestor's psychological inheritance in an informed way. The psychological genealogy we suspect or uncover can be shared with family and can inform health professionals.[27]

My hope is that family historians will increasingly uncover and share not only their family stories, and local and social history, but consider and share their family's possible psychological inheritance as well. We are in a privileged position. So much more is known about mental health, mental disability, mental distress, and how the effects of insecure attachment, adversity, and trauma might be reversed. Many of us are fortunate not to live in a culture that routinely silences those who struggle emotionally. Many can access evidence-based self-help, and "find the places, the spaces, and the people that fit who we really are and allow us to live our best lives" (DePaulo 2016; Castañón 2020). Others share what they learn about their family with a therapist. However we choose to use our deepening understanding of our ancestors, we can remember the "past does not have to define . . . us, 'it can empower us'" (Evans 2021, p. 98) The insight we gain can give living family new opportunities to thrive and pass on a healthier psychological legacy.

Funding: This research received no external funding.

Acknowledgments: Consultant George Regkoukos; external reviewer: Debanjali Biswas.

Conflicts of Interest: The author declares no conflict of interest.

Notes

1. As Asmussen et al outlines in "Adverse Childhood Experiences" (Asmussen et al. 2020).
2. The work of Hinrichs et al. noted the five personality styles are not exclusive to adult children of alcoholics (Hinrichs et al. 2011): pp. 487–98.
3. Defining the Traits of Dysfunctional Families, King University Online (2017). *King University Online.* https://online.king.edu/news/dysfunctional-families/ (accessed on 12 October 2021).
4. See the impact sudies of ACEs in "How Aces Affect Health" (2021) https://centerforyouthwellness.org/health-impacts/#:~:text=Experiencing%204%20or%20more%20ACEs,%2C%20diabetes%2C%20Alzheimers%20and%20suicide (accessed on 12 October 2021); Felitti et al. "Childhood Abuse and Household Dysfunction" (Felitti et al. 2019).
5. "Experiencing Childhood Trauma Makes Body and Brain Age Faster: Findings Could Help Explain Why Children Who Suffer Trauma Often Face Poor Health Later in Life". *Sciencedaily.* (2020) American Psychological Association. https://www.sciencedaily.com/releases/2020/08/200803092120.htm (accessed on 12 October 2021).
6. "Who Do You Think You Are?", (2004). TV programme. BBC 2: BBC.
7. From an interview with Phyllis Mary Skells, née Woods, known as Mary (2015).

8   Phyllis Mary Skells, née Woods, known as Mary and Frances Irene Pell née Woods, known as Rene (2014).
9   As indicated in the study paper (Risks to Mental Health: An Overview of Vulnerabilities and Risk Factors 2012) published by the World Health Organization.
10   Turner et al. (2018) showed that alcohol use disorder is predated by either anxiety or depression in 45 per cent of sufferers.
11   (Genetics and Epigenetics of Addiction Drugfacts | National Institute on Drug Abuse 2019). *National Institute on Drug Abuse.* https://www.drugabuse.gov/publications/drugfacts/genetics-epigenetics-addiction (accessed on 12 October 2021).
12   Causes of Death in England and Wales, 1851–1860 to 1891–1900: The Decennial Supplements http://doc.ukdataservice.ac.uk/doc/3552/mrdoc/pdf/guide.pdf (accessed on 12 October 2021).
13   The head of the boys' school also lost two children, including his daughter Ethel May Law, aged 17 years, when Walter was aged ten.
14   For example, Peterborough Standard-Saturday 6 January 1900. 1900. "Thorney: Parish Register", p. 8, column 3. 1900. Thorney Abbey Girls Logbook 1863–1895, C/ES155AS, 4 October 1895, p. 398.
15   The Canadian Homestead Act gave 160 acres for free to any male farmer who agreed to cultivate at least 40 acres and to build a permanent dwelling within three years. The only cost to the farmer being a $10 administration fee. This condition of "proving up the homestead" was instituted to prevent speculators from gaining control of the land. Congress, Homestead, Homestead Congress, and View profile. 2010. "The Canadian Homestead Act". *Homesteadcongress.Blogspot.Com.* http://homesteadcongress.blogspot.com/2010/12/canadian-homestead-act.html (accessed on 12 October 2021).
16   As told to me by his son-in-law Harry Drabble and his niece Phyllis Mary Skells. The original tenancy book is in the author's keeping.
17   According to Walter and Hilda's marriage certificate Hilda was a housekeeper residing at 38 High Oaks Road, Welwyn Garden City [AL8 7BS]. This property was estimated value of estimated value of £1,137,202 in June 2021.
18   Twenty-nine years was the average age of woman at their first birth in 1928, in Thompson et al. (2012) Olympic Britain.
19   At this stage in their life, children often show a fear of strangers and are clearly more anxious when they are separated from their key attachment figure. However, some babies show stranger fear and separation anxiety much more frequently and intensely than others. Could such a pattern of behavior reflect the changes in the brain that Hendrix et al. (2021) discovered in infants whose mothers had been emotionally neglected in their childhood?
20   *Sheffield Daily Telegraph.* "War-time Population" (21.10.39), p. 4.
21   *Sheffield Daily Telegraph.* "Parents Prefer Family at Home" (1939) p. 6.; (The Evacuated Children of the Second World War 2021) *Imperial War Museums.* [Accessed 18 October 2021]. url: https://www.iwm.org.uk/history/the-evacuated-children-of-the-second-world-war (accessed on 12 October 2021).
22   "The Original Promise and Law". *World Association of Girl Guides and Girl Scouts.* url: https://www.wagggs.org/en/about-us/our-history/original-promise-and-law/ (accessed on 12 October 2021).
23   Interview with Sheila Cousins née Gough, Doreen's closest friend c1954–1974. In person and Facebook message. (2021)
24   Interview with Sheila Cousins. (2021); Schumann and Orehek. "Avoidant and Defensive" (Schumann and Orehek 2017).
25   Interview with Sheila Cousins. (2021).
26   Conversations with my mother and father. Interview with Sheila Cousins. (2021).
27   A guide to mood and depressive disorders enables the creation of a mental health family-tree. See https://www.familyaware.org/help-someone/create-a-mental-health-family-tree (2020) (accessed on 12 October 2021).

References

Ainsworth, Mary D. Salter, and Silvia M. Bell. 1970. Attachment, Exploration, and Separation: Illustrated by the Behavior of One-Year-Olds in a Strange Situation. *Child Development* 41: 49–67. [CrossRef]

Asmussen, Kirsten, Freyja Fischer, Elaine Drayton, and Tom McBride. 2020. Adverse Childhood Experiences What We Know, What We Don't Know, and What Should Happen Next. *Early Intervention Foundation.* Available online: https://www.eif.org.uk/report/adverse-childhood-experiences-what-we-know-what-we-dont-know-and-what-should-happen-next (accessed on 12 October 2021).

Ballard, Mary E. 1993. Adult children of alcoholics: Security, avoidance, and ambivalence in attachment to parents. Paper presented at the Meeting of the Society for Research in Child Development, New Orleans, LA, USA, March 25–28; Available online: https://files.eric.ed.gov/fulltext/ED357312.pdf (accessed on 12 October 2021).

Barnett, Lynn James, and Joyce Robertson. 1991. *Separation and the Very Young.* London: Free Association Books.

Beiner, Guy. 2014. Probing the Boundaries of Irish Memory: From Postmemory to Prememory and Back. *Irish Historical Studies* 39: 302–303. [CrossRef]

Beletsis, Susan G., and Stephanie Brown. 1981. A developmental framework for understanding the adult children of alcoholics. *Journal of Addictions and Health* 2: 187–203.

Blair-Gómez, Carolina. 2013. The Biological Basis of Parent-Infant Attachment: Foundations and Implications for Further Development. *Informes Psicológicos* 13: 23–40.

Boelen, Paul A., Maarten C. Eisma, Geert E. Smid, and Lonneke IM Lenferink. 2020. Prolonged grief disorder in section II of DSM-5: A commentary. *European Journal of Psychotraumatology* 11: 1771008. [CrossRef] [PubMed]

Boulware, Dessirae L., and Ngoc H. Bui. 2016. Bereaved African American adults: The role of social support, religious coping, and continuing bonds. *Journal of Loss and Trauma* 21: 192–202. [CrossRef]

Carvallo, Mauricio, and Shira Gabriel. 2020. No Man is an Island: People Who Say They don't Need Other People Actually Care about Close Relationships | SPSP. Available online: https://www.spsp.org/news-center/blog/carvallo-gabriel-dismissive-avoidants-belonging (accessed on 12 October 2021).

Castañón, Laura Childhood Trauma Changes Your Brain. 2020. But it doesn't Have to be Permanent. News@Northeastern. Available online: https://news.northeastern.edu/2020/02/20/childhood-trauma-changes-your-brain-but-it-doesnt-have-to-be-permanent/ (accessed on 12 October 2021).

Cobbe, Frances P. 1878. Wife torture in England. *The Contemporary Review* 32: 69.

Colich, Natalie L., Maya L. Rosen, Eileen S. Williams, and Katie A. McLaughlin. 2020. Biological aging in childhood and adolescence following experiences of threat and deprivation: A systematic review and meta-analysis. *Psychological Bulletin* 146: 721. [CrossRef] [PubMed]

Connors, Mary E. 1997. The Renunciation of Love: Dismissive Attachment and Its Treatment. *Psychoanalytic Psychology* 14: 475–93. [CrossRef]

Craddock, Gerald, Cormac Doran, and Larry McNutt, eds. 2018. *Transforming Our World through Design, Diversity and Education: Proceedings of Universal Design and Higher Education in Transformation Congress*. Amsterdam: IOS Press, vols. 256.

DePaulo, Bella. 2016. Psychologist Reveals Science Behind a Fulfilling Single Life. *American Psychological Association*. Available online: https://www.apa.org (accessed on 12 October 2021).

Duschinsky, Robbie. 2020. *Cornerstones of Attachment Research*. Oxford: Oxford University Press.

Edelstein, Robin S., and Phillip R. Shaver. 2004. Avoidant attachment: Exploration of an oxymoron. In *Handbook of Closeness and Intimacy*. Hove: Psychology Press, pp. 407–22.

Elsevier. 2021. Childhood Neglect Leaves Generational Imprint: Distinct Neural Connectivity Found in the Babies of Mothers Who Experienced Neglect as Children. *ScienceDaily*. Available online: www.sciencedaily.com/releases/2021/01/210119085222.htm (accessed on 12 October 2021).

Evans, Tanya. 2021. How Do Family Historians Work with Memory? *Journal of Family History* 46: 92–106. [CrossRef]

Fearon, Pasco. 2004. Comments on Turton Et Al: On the Complexities of Trauma, Loss and the Intergenerational Transmission of Disorganized Relationships. *Attachment & Human Development* 6: 255–61. [CrossRef]

Feeney, Brooke C., Jude Cassidy, and Fatima Ramos-Marcuse. 2008. The Generalization of Attachment Representations to New Social Situations: Predicting Behavior during Initial Interactions with Strangers. *Journal of Personality and Social Psychology* 95: 1481–98. [CrossRef]

Felitti, Vincent J. 2002. The relationship of adverse childhood experiences to adult health: Turning gold into lead/Belastungen in der Kindheit und Gesundheit im Erwachsenenalter: Die Verwandlung von Gold in Blei. *Zeitschrift für Psychosomatische Medizin und Psychotherapie* 48: 359–69. [CrossRef] [PubMed]

Felitti, Vincent J., Robert F. Anda, Dale Nordenberg, David F. Williamson, Alison M. Spitz, Valerie Edwards, Mary P. Koss, and James S. Marks. 2019. Reprint of: Relationship of childhood abuse and household dysfunction to many of the leading causes of death in adults: The adverse childhood experiences (ACE) study. *American Journal of Preventive Medicine* 56: 774–86. [CrossRef] [PubMed]

Firestone, Lisa. 2013. How Your Attachment Style Affects Your Parenting. *Psychology Today*. Available online: https://www.psychologytoday.com/us/blog/compassion-matters/201510/how-your-attachment-style-affects-your-parenting (accessed on 12 October 2021).

Fraga, Juli. 2018. Learn Your Own Attachment Style to Become a Better Parent | Aeon Essays. *Aeon*. Available online: https://aeon.co/essays/learn-your-own-attachment-style-to-become-a-better-parent (accessed on 12 October 2021).

Fraley, R. Chris, and Phillip R. Shaver. 1997. Adult attachment and the suppression of unwanted thoughts. *Journal of Personality and Social Psychology* 73: 1080–91. [CrossRef]

Fraley, R. Chris, and Phillip R. Shaver. 2000. Adult romantic attachment: Theoretical developments, emerging controversies, and unanswered questions. *Review of General Psychology* 4: 132–54. [CrossRef]

Genetics and Epigenetics of Addiction Drugfacts | National Institute on Drug Abuse. 2019. National Institute on Drug Abuse. Available online: https://www.drugabuse.gov/publications/drugfacts/genetics-epigenetics-addiction (accessed on 12 October 2021).

Gillies, James, and Robert A. Neimeyer. 2006. Loss, Grief, and the Search for Significance: Toward a Model of Meaning Reconstruction in Bereavement. *Journal of Constructivist Psychology* 19: 31–65. [CrossRef]

Griffin, Emma. 2020. *Bread Winner: An Intimate History of the Victorian Economy*. New Haven and London: Yale University Press.

Grossmann, Karin. 1989. Avoidance as a communicative strategy in attachment relationships. Paper presented at the Fourth World Congress for Infant Psychiatry and Allied Disciplines, Lugano, Switzerland, September 20–24.

Hendrix, Cassandra L., Daniel D. Dilks, Brooke G. McKenna, Anne L. Dunlop, Elizabeth J. Corwin, and Patricia A. Brennan. 2021. Maternal Childhood Adversity Associates with Frontoamygdala Connectivity in Neonates. *Biological Psychiatry: Cognitive Neuroscience and Neuroimaging* 6: 470–78. [CrossRef]

Hinrichs, Jonathan, Jared DeFife, and Drew Westen. 2011. Personality Subtypes in Adolescent and Adult Children of Alcoholics. *Journal of Nervous & Mental Disease* 199: 487–98. [CrossRef]

Hirsch, Marianne. 2008. The generation of postmemory. *Poetics Today* 29: 103–28. [CrossRef]

Huberman, Michael, and Chris Minns. 2007. The times they are not changin': Days and hours of work in Old and New Worlds, 1870–2000. *Explorations in Economic History* 44: 538–67. [CrossRef]

Iyengar, Udita, Purva Rajhans, Peter Fonagy, Lane Strathearn, and Sohye Kim. 2019. Unresolved Trauma and Reorganization in Mothers: Attachment and Neuroscience Perspectives. *Frontiers in Psychology* 10: 1–9. [CrossRef]

Jarrett, Christian. 2019. First Study to Investigate How Attachment Style Changes through Multiple Decades of Life. Research Digest. Available online: https://digest.bps.org.uk/2019/05/09/first-study-to-investigate-how-attachment-style-changes-through-multiple-decades-of-life/ (accessed on 12 October 2021).

Joinson, Carla. 2018. Prairie Madness | Healing, Hell, and the History of American Insane Asylums. Available online: https://hhhasylum.com/tag/prairie-madness/ (accessed on 12 October 2021).

Kelley, Michelle L., Valarie M. Schroeder, Cathy G. Cooke, Leslie Gumienny, Amanda Jeffrey Platter, and William Fals-Stewart. 2010. Mothers' Versus Fathers' Alcohol Abuse and Attachment in Adult Daughters of Alcoholics. *Journal of Family Issues* 31: 1555–70. [CrossRef]

Khodabakhsh, Mohammadreza. 2012. Attachment styles as predictors of empathy in nursing students. *Journal of Medical Ethics and History of Medicine* 5: 1–7.

Kim, Sohye, Peter Fonagy, Jon Allen, and Lane Strathearn. 2014. Mothers' Unresolved Trauma Blunts Amygdala Response to Infant Distress. *Social Neuroscience* 9: 352–63. [CrossRef]

Kirmayer, Laurence J., Gregory M. Brass, and Caroline L. Tait. 2000. The mental health of Aboriginal peoples: Transformations of identity and community. *The Canadian Journal of Psychiatry* 45: 607–16. [CrossRef]

Kokou-Kpolou, Cyrille Kossigan, Sunyoung Park, Lonneke IM Lenferink, Steven Kotar Iorfa, Manuel Fernández-Alcántara, Daniel Derivois, and Jude Mary Cénat. 2021. Prolonged grief and depression: A latent class analysis. *Psychiatry Research* 299: 113864. [CrossRef] [PubMed]

Lai, Carlo, Massimiliano Luciani, Federico Galli, Emanuela Morelli, Roberta Cappelluti, Italo Penco, Paola Aceto, and Luigi Lombardo. 2015. Attachment style dimensions can affect prolonged grief risk in caregivers of terminally ill patients with cancer. *American Journal of Hospice and Palliative Medicine* 32: 855–60. [CrossRef]

Landsberg, Alison. 2009. Memory, empathy, and the politics of identification. *International Journal of Politics, Culture, and Society* 22: 221–9. [CrossRef]

Langhamer, Claire. 2013. *The English in Love: The Intimate Story of an Emotional Revolution*, 1st ed. Oxford: Oxford University Press.

Lanzoni, Susan. 2015. A Short History of Empathy. The Atlantic. Available online: https://www.theatlantic.com/health/archive/2015/10/a-short-history-of-empathy/409912/ (accessed on 12 October 2021).

Lapping, Claudia. 2019. Mourning and Melancholia. In *The Routledge Handbook of Psychoanalytic Political Theory*. Edited by Yannis Stavrakakis. London and New York: Routledge, pp. 208–20.

Lovett, Joan. 2014. *Trauma-Attachment Tangle: Modifying Emdr to Help Children Resolve Trauma and Develop Loving Relationships*. New York and London: Routledge.

Lupien, Sonia J., Sophie Parent, Alan C. Evans, Richard E. Tremblay, Philip David Zelazo, Vincent Corbo, Jens C. Pruessner, and Jean R. Séguin. 2011. Larger amygdala but no change in hippocampal volume in 10-year-old children exposed to maternal depressive symptomatology since birth. *Proceedings of the National Academy of Sciences* 108: 14324–9. [CrossRef]

Maccallum, Fiona, and Richard A. Bryant. 2018. Prolonged Grief and Attachment Security: A Latent Class Analysis. *Psychiatry Research* 268: 297–302. [CrossRef]

McEwen, Bruce S., and Huda Akil. 2020. Revisiting the stress concept: Implications for affective disorders. *Journal of Neuroscience* 40: 12–21. [CrossRef]

McIntosh, Tania. 1997. A Price Must Be Paid for Motherhood: The Experience of Maternity in Sheffield, 1879–1939. Ph.D. dissertation, University of Sheffield, Sheffield, UK.

Mikulincer, Mario, and Victor Florian. 1998. The relationship between adult attachment styles and emotional and cognitive reactions to stressful events. In *Attachment Theory and Close Relationships*. Edited by Jeffry A. Simpson and William SE. Rholes. New York: Guilford Press, pp. 143–65.

Mikulincer, Mario, and Phillip R. Shaver. 2003. The attachment behavioral system in adulthood: Activation, psychodynamics, and interpersonal processes. In *Advances in Experimental Social Psychology*. Edited by Mark P. Zanna. San Diego: Academic Press, vols. 35, pp. 53–152.

Moore, Susan, Doreen Rosenthal, and Rebecca Robinson. 2020. *The Psychology of Family History: Exploring Our Genealogy*. London and New York: Routledge.

Nickerson, Angela, Richard A. Bryant, Idan M. Aderka, Devon E. Hinton, and Stefan G. Hofmann. 2013. The impacts of parental loss and adverse parenting on mental health: Findings from the National Comorbidity Survey-Replication. *Psychological Trauma: Theory, Research, Practice, and Policy* 5: 119–27. [CrossRef]

Parker-Drabble, Helen. 2020. *Who Do I Think You Were? A Victorian's Inheritance*. London: Animi Press.

Prescott, Carol A., Steven H. Aggen, and Kenneth S. Kendler. 2000. Sex-specific genetic influences on the comorbidity of alcoholism and major depression in a population-based sample of US twins. *Archives of General Psychiatry* 57: 803–11. [CrossRef] [PubMed]

Qin, Shaozheng, Christina B. Young, Xujun Duan, Tianwen Chen, Kaustubh Supekar, and Vinod Menon. 2014. Amygdala Subregional Structure and Intrinsic Functional Connectivity Predicts Individual Differences in Anxiety During Early Childhood. *Biological Psychiatry* 75: 892–900. [CrossRef] [PubMed]

Reisz, Samantha, Robbie Duschinsky, and Daniel J. Siegel. 2018. Disorganized attachment and defense: Exploring John Bowlby's unpublished reflections. *Attachment & Human Development* 20: 107–34. [CrossRef]

Risks to Mental Health: An Overview of Vulnerabilities and Risk Factors–Background Paper by WHO Secretariat for the Development of a Comprehensive Mental Health Action Plan. 2012. Geneva: World Health Organization, Available online: https://www.who.int/mental_health/mhgap/risks_to_mental_health_EN_27_08_12.pdf (accessed on 12 October 2021).

Rollero, Chiara, and Norma De Piccoli. 2010. Place attachment, identification and environment perception: An empirical study. *Journal of Environmental Psychology* 30: 198–205. [CrossRef]

Saatcioglu, Omer, Rahsan Erim, and Durcan Cakmak. 2006. Role of Family in Alcohol and Substance Abuse. *Psychiatry and Clinical Neurosciences* 60: 125–32. [CrossRef]

Saphire-Bernstein, Shimon, Baldwin. M. Way, Heejung S. Kim, David K. Sherman, and Shelley E. Taylor. 2011. Oxytocin Receptor Gene (OXTR) Is Related to Psychological Resources. *Proceedings of the National Academy of Sciences* 108: 15118–22. [CrossRef]

Schindler, Andreas. 2019. Attachment and substance use disorders—theoretical models, empirical evidence, and implications for treatment. *Frontiers in Psychiatry* 10: 727. [CrossRef] [PubMed]

Schumann, Karina, and Edward Orehek. 2017. Avoidant and Defensive: Adult Attachment and Quality of Apologies. *Journal of Social and Personal Relationships* 36: 809–33. [CrossRef]

Seymour, Susan. 2013. It Takes a Village to Raise a Child: Attachment Theory and Multiple Childcare in Alor, Indonesia, and in North India. In *Attachment Reconsidered: Cultural Perspectives on A Western Theory*. New York: Palgrave Macmillan, pp. 115–39.

Shaver, Phillip R., and Cindy Hazan. 1993. Adult romantic attachment: Theory and evidence. In *Advances in Personal Relationships*. Edited by Daniel Perlman and Warren Jones. London: Jessica Kingsley, vols. 4, pp. 29–70.

Shaw, Emma. 2020. "Who We Are, And Why We Do It": A Demographic Overview and The Cited Motivations of Australia's Family Historians. *Journal of Family History* 45: 109–24. [CrossRef]

Simpson, Jeffry A., and Jay Belsky. 2008. Attachment Theory within a Modern Evolutionary Framework: Theory, Research, and Clinical Applications. In *Handbook of Attachment: Theory, Research, And Clinical Applications*. Edited by Jude Cassidy and Phillip R. Shaver. New York: Guilford, pp. 91–116.

Solomon, Andrew. 2001. *The Noonday Demon: An Atlas of Depression*. New York: Scribner.

Sochos, Antigonos, and Sadia Aleem. 2021. Parental Attachment Style and Young Persons' Adjustment to Bereavement. In *Child & Youth Care Forum*. New York and Philadelphia: Springer US, pp. 1–19.

Sotero, Michelle. 2006. A Conceptual Model of Historical Trauma: Implications for Public Health Practice and Research. *Journal of Health Disparities Research and Practice* 1: 93–108.

Strange, Julie-Marie. 2006. Dangerous Motherhood: Insanity and Childbirth in Victorian Britain by Hilary Marland. *History* 91: 471. [CrossRef]

Strange, Julie-Marie. 2012. Fatherhood, Providing, And Attachment in Late Victorian and Edwardian Working-Class Families. *The Historical Journal* 55: 1007–27. [CrossRef]

Taggart, Geoff, and Jo Elsey. 2021. Supervision and Adult Attachment. Available online: https://tactyc.org.uk/pdfs/Taggart%20and%20Elsey.pdf (accessed on 12 October 2021).

The Evacuated Children of the Second World War. 2021. Imperial War Museums. Available online: https://www.iwm.org.uk/history/the-evacuated-children-of-the-second-world-war (accessed on 12 October 2021).

Thompson, Gavin, Oliver Hawkins, Aliyah Dar, and Mark Taylor. 2012. Olympic Britain: Social and economic change since the 1908 and 1948 London Games. *Retrieved October* 1: 2014.

Turan, Numan, William T. Hoyt, and Özgür Erdur-Baker. 2016. Gender, attachment orientations, rumination, and symptomatic distress: Test of a moderated mediation model. *Personality and Individual Differences* 102: 234–9. [CrossRef]

Turner, Sarah, Natalie Mota, James Bolton, and Jitender Sareen. 2018. Self-medication with alcohol or drugs for mood and anxiety disorders: A narrative review of the epidemiological literature. *Depression and Anxiety* 35: 851–60. [CrossRef]

Vaillant, George E. 2009. *Natural History of Alcoholism*, 2nd ed. Revisited. Cambridge: Harvard University Press.

Voges, Juané, Astrid Berg, and Dana J. H. Niehaus. 2019. Revisiting the African Origins of Attachment Research—50 Years on From Ainsworth: A Descriptive Review. *Infant Mental Health Journal* 40: 799–816. [CrossRef]

Vungkhanching, Martha, Kenneth J. Sher, Kristina M. Jackson, and Gilbert R. Parra. 2004. Relation of Attachment Style to Family History of Alcoholism and Alcohol Use Disorders in Early Adulthood. *Drug and Alcohol Dependence* 75: 47–53. [CrossRef]

Wegscheider, Sharon. 1981. *Another Chance: Hope and Health for the Alcoholic Family*, 1st ed. Palo Alto: Science and Behavior Books.

West, Malcolm L., and Adrienne E. R. Keller. 1991. Parentification of the child: A case study of Bowlby's compulsive care-giving attachment pattern. *American Journal of Psychotherapy* 45: 425–31. [CrossRef]

Womersley, Kate, Katherine Ripullone, and Jane Elizabeth Hirst. 2021. Tackling inequality in maternal health: Beyond the postpartum. *Future Healthcare Journal* 8: 31. [CrossRef] [PubMed]

Yehuda, Rachel, and Amy Lehrner. 2018. Intergenerational Transmission of Trauma Effects: Putative Role of Epigenetic Mechanisms. *World Psychiatry* 17: 243–57. [CrossRef]

Zelekha, Yaron, and Erez Yaakobi. 2020. Intergenerational Attachment Orientations: Gender Differences and Environmental Contribution. *PLoS ONE* 15: e0233906. [CrossRef]

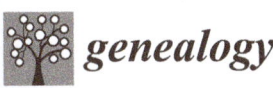 *genealogy*

Article

The Effects of DNA Test Results on Biological and Family Identities

Catherine Agnes Theunissen

Independent Researcher, Auckland 1010, New Zealand; catherine.a.theunissen@gmail.com

Abstract: Direct-to-consumer DNA testing is increasingly affordable and accessible, and the potential implications from these tests are becoming more important. As additional people partake in DNA testing, larger population groups and information will cause further refinement of results and more extensive databases, resulting in further potential opportunities to connect biological relatives and increased chances of testers potentially having their identities re-aligned, reinforced or solidified. The effects of DNA testing were explored through 16 semi-structured in-depth interviews conducted with participants who had received their DNA test results. These participants came from diverse groups, genders and ethnic backgrounds. A thematic analysis found that notions of family were frequently challenged with unexpected DNA test results causing shifts in personal and social identities, especially in their family and biological identities. Discrepancies in DNA test results prompted re-negotiation of these identities and affected their feelings of belonging to their perceived social groups. Participants' identities were important to them in varying degrees, with some feeling stronger connections with specific identities, thus having significant re-alignment of these identities and feelings of belonging. This article discusses the thematic analysis's findings and explores how identities of the participants, many of whom took the test for genealogical purposes, were affected by DNA test results. As more people undertake DNA testing, it is important to explore how it may change the notions of family in the future and how their biological and family identities are affected.

Keywords: biological identity; family identity; DNA testing; thematic analysis; biogeographic ancestry

Citation: Theunissen, Catherine Agnes. 2022. The Effects of DNA Test Results on Biological and Family Identities. *Genealogy* 6: 17. https://doi.org/10.3390/genealogy6010017

Received: 2 December 2021
Accepted: 13 February 2022
Published: 17 February 2022

Publisher's Note: MDPI stays neutral with regard to jurisdictional claims in published maps and institutional affiliations.

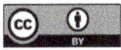

Copyright: © 2022 by the author. Licensee MDPI, Basel, Switzerland. This article is an open access article distributed under the terms and conditions of the Creative Commons Attribution (CC BY) license (https:// creativecommons.org/licenses/by/ 4.0/).

1. Introduction

Direct-to-consumer (DTC) genetic testing is becoming more pervasive as people complete tests to find out more about themselves. Evidently, according to Jhamb (2021), the DTC testing industry is projected to "grow from $1.4 billion in 2020 to $2.6 billion by 2025 with a compound annual growth rate (CAGR) of 14.2% for the period of 2020–2025" (para. 1). This reinforces the growth of the industry and reflects the increase in testing (namely, autosomal, mtDNA and Y-DNA), where the implications from people receiving their results are becoming more complex and, in some cases, changing people's lives. Therefore, exploring the potential implications and effects for people considering taking a test is becoming increasingly important, especially as databases grow and further developments and refinements are made.

This article discusses selected findings from a qualitative research study that interviewed sixteen participants on the effects of DNA tests on their identities. Interviews were semi-structured and in-depth, and the interview data were analysed using thematic analysis. Participants were found through a combination of purposive and snowball sampling, and they had to have completed a DNA test or would be receiving their results during the time of data collection.

The study found that notions of family were frequently challenged, with unexpected DNA test results causing shifts in personal and social identities. This was especially prevalent in family and biological identities, which conforms to views such as that of molecular biologist Bernath (2015), who observed the linkages between social identity and biological identity. Bernath (2015) claimed that in the last 20 years, the term 'DNA' has become synonymous with identity. The current study also found that discrepancies in DNA test results prompted re-negotiation of these identities and affected feelings of belonging to their perceived social groups (primarily family and biological groups, which will be the focus of this article). Depending on the importance of their identities, participants who attached stronger significance to specific identities and whose identities were challenged had significant re-alignments of their identities and feelings of belonging when these ideals were challenged.

Identity is a multifaceted concept that has been widely defined and redefined. Although the concept of identity has been explored by a multitude of scholars since Socrates, the term 'identity' was not coined until John Locke (1632–1704) first mentioned 'personal identity' (Coulmas 2019; Izenberg 2016). Much later, in the mid-20th century, 'identity' was popularised by Erik Erikson to describe different forms of identities (Coulmas 2019; Fearon 1999; Harvard University n.d.; Izenberg 2016). While recognising the development of the term, this article focuses on identity as a combination of identities, following the notion that identity is an ongoing process where one adapts to their mutable environmental conditions (Coulmas 2019). This includes the three dimensions of 'self' being closely linked with one's identity, which includes the bodily self (own desires and wishes), relational self (from social and cultural interaction) and the reflective self (where one can observe oneself and relationships) (Izenberg 2016).

Although participants in the current study did not need to specify their type of DNA testing conducted, some participants elaborated on details that were specific to certain types of testing. Many frequently used terms such as 'ethnicity estimates', which are connected to autosomal DNA tests, whereas other participants mentioned specifically looking at their direct paternal or maternal lineages. Thus, to provide context, genetic testing types and DNA tests are introduced, along with five key well-known commercial companies that offer the tests that participants had likely taken. Additionally, although there is a substantial body of knowledge addressing social group identities, Tajfel and Turner's social identity theory is briefly introduced to provide context for key aspects of identity identified by participants.

2. Genetic Testing Types

Genetic testing is available in multiple forms, and depending on the purpose of the testing, different tests will yield different results. Genetic testing is conducted by analysing a sample of blood or body tissue (Anzilotti 2021). In the case of DTC tests, these are usually done through a saliva sample, either by spitting into a tube or using a swab. Since the completion of the Human Genome Project in 2003 (National Human Genome Research Institute 2018), DNA tests have become cheaper and easier to access, resulting in further developments. The three main types that participants took included Y-DNA/Y chromosome testing, mtDNA/mitochondrial testing and autosomal testing.

Y-DNA testing only focuses on the paternal line, whereas mtDNA testing looks at the maternal line (van Oven et al. 2013; Schneider et al. 2019). Schneider et al. (2019) explained that markers located on the Y chromosome were only passed from father to son, which reflected the geographical origin of a male's ancestors. mtDNA, however, is passed down from mothers to sons and daughters, allowing any sex to take the test (van Oven and Kayser 2008). mtDNA testing uses "sequential accumulation of mutations along maternally inherited lineages, which can be represented in a tree reflecting the phylogenetic relationships of known mtDNA variants", which help identify one's maternal lineage (van Oven and Kayser 2008, p. 387). However, a limitation of these tests are that by only focusing on the Y chromosomes and mtDNA polymorphisms, the tests will only trace back through the particular lineages and not the 16,383 ancestors from up to fourteen generations ago that the person is related to in equal measure (Elliott and Brodwin 2002). Nevertheless, these two tests provide potential 'matches' with genetic cousins and a haplogroup assignment indicating the person's placement on the Y-chromosome or mtDNA haplotree.

The third test, the autosomal DNA test, looks at a selection of markers scattered across a person's entire genome and provides matches with genetic relatives from the person's ancestral lines. These tests also provide a biogeographical ancestry estimate based on comparisons with reference populations (Anderson 2021). However, as Schneider et al. (2019) pointed out, the markers located on the autosomes are inherited from both parents and, therefore, reflect the geographic origins of both. They explained that autosomal DNA is reassorted in each generation so that "only half of autosomal DNA markers are still present in each off-spring" (Schneider et al. 2019, p. 877). When biological ancestors come from different regions, autosomal DNA markers can be used to make 'quantitative inferences' about a person's mixed biological ancestry (Schneider et al. 2019). Dooney (2017) wrote that DNA specialist Brad Argent detailed that, as genetic material is passed down from person to person, it can become diluted, especially in a world where people are increasingly diverse.

The further apart the geographic origins of two people are, the greater the differences will be (Schneider et al. 2019). These also reflect migration, where certain DNA markers are seen in particular population groups in specific regions or have commonalities with population groups in certain regions. Due to most human populations having migrated many times throughout history, thereby mixing with nearby groups, the "ethnicity estimates based on genetic testing may differ from an individual's expectations" (Medline Plus 2020, para. 5). Nonetheless, the possibility of different combinations of DNA from the same parents creates complexity and has more possibilities for those using their DNA test results to connect with biological relatives. These forms of testing can be used for DTC tests, where individuals can do a test to gain more information about their ancestry (Best Tests 2014).

Although some participants questioned the validity of the frequently changing ethnicity estimates, they were confident about close matches through centimorgans (cM). The DTC autosomal tests estimate the closeness of relationships through the use of cM. The more DNA is shared, the higher the cM becomes. Therefore, relatives with high cM are likely to be more closely linked (Darroch and Smith 2021). This is reflected with 'matches', where testers will be connected to those with a high proportion of shared genetic material (Strand and Källén 2021). The DTC company 23andMe launched the 'relative finding' feature, which used autosomal DNA to show both lines, rather than one's paternal or maternal lineage; soon after, FamilyTreeDNA launched their 'family finder' in 2010 (Darroch and Smith 2021). Since then, multiple DTC companies expanded their markets and now offer various tests.

Genetic testing is, however, not free of controversy. Elliott and Brodwin (2002) stated that genetic information was given too much authority in deciding questions about identity. One's genetic ancestry might not reflect one's identity, they wrote. However, they also pointed out that even though genetic testing could disrupt identity claims, it could corroborate such claims and confirm origin stories, family history or rights to group membership. Argent (as cited in Dooney 2017) added, "[w]e are shaped by the stories of our ancestors, and not necessarily by our genes" (para. 19). In a similar vein, Lawton and Foeman (2017) stated that AncestryDNA was pushing people to the edge of their biogeographical ancestry classifications, giving additional information on how they identified themselves and included a range of factors such as "phenotype, social class, languages spoken, family narratives, and peer relations" (p. 80). Nevertheless, while consumers might be pushed to the edge of biogeographic ancestral classifications, a weakness in DNA testing remains where regions such as Africa, Asia and the Pacific are still under-represented (Dooney 2017) due to many DTC testers being based in other regions and datasets not yet being large or accurate enough in these under-represented areas. However, this may change as testing becomes more popular, accessible and cheaper. As more people take the tests, larger and seemingly more accurate databases are created that will help refine features such as 'ethnicity estimates' and better represent currently under-represented regions. DNA testing can also continue to help those who were separated during wars and conflicts or through adoptions, similarly to an experience described by Puig et al. (2019). Puig et al. (2019) detailed how mtDNA testing helped a man find his maternal line and allowed him to reconnect with his family after many decades of separation. This man was one of many people evacuated to Belgium during the Spanish Civil War, and was then adopted into a new family and had his name changed. He was unable to remember his childhood, and DNA testing provided him with the tool to find his biological family.

3. Commercial Tests Offered

There are currently five commonly used and well-known DNA companies, namely, AncestryDNA, MyHeritage, FamilyTreeDNA, 23andME and LivingDNA. AncestryDNA (n.d.) offers a DNA test that connects one to relatives and offers ethnicity estimates based on over 1500 regions. Since this study's completion in 2020, AncestryDNA (n.d.) started offering a 'traits' test in the Australasian market, where one can additionally discover biological traits shown in their DNA. MyHeritage (n.d.) offers testing to identify ethnic origins and new relatives. They claim to have a DNA database of 5.4 million people. FamilyTreeDNA offers family ancestry testing, connecting testers with their autosomal DNA relatives within the last five generations and providing a breakdown of origins and where each DNA segment comes from (Gene by Gene, Ltd. n.d.)Gene by Gene, Ltd. Furthermore, they offer mtDNA and Y-DNA testing, which allow the user to be matched with genetic relatives in the databases. (23andMe, Inc. n.d.) offers two main types of testing: 'Ancestry + Traits Service' and 'Health + Ancestry Service'. The first focuses on a person's origins, DNA relatives and 30+ trait reports; the latter test details everything from the first test with additional health predispositions, wellness and carrier status reports. In addition to this, they also include a family health history tree and provide insights into the tester's health based on genetic data. Lastly, similarly to AncestryDNA, LivingDNA Ltd. (n.d.) offers an 'ancestry kit', where the testing shows recent ancestry, sub-regional breakdowns, DNA matching and extended ancestry in one test. This test includes mtDNA and Y-DNA haplogroup reports (haplotypes are found within a haplogroup and are based on DNA information from a mtDNA or Y-DNA test, where specific markers, mutations and variations indicate one's haplotype relationships and help predict a haplogroup, King and Jobling 2009). They also offer a secondary test, which includes an ancestry test with wellbeing, giving additional details on vitamin response, food metabolism and nutrition, exercise and recovery based on the tester's genetic makeup. Tests are region-dependent and are not all available globally. Thus, participants did not always refer to all available tests. They did, however, describe (intergroup) behaviours that demonstrated similarities, which they linked to having a biological connection through DNA.

4. Intergroup Behaviours and Social Identity Theory

Intergroup behaviours and the connection with social identity are prevalent in understanding participants' feelings of belonging, group membership and the joining of these aspects to their identities. In the early 1970s, British social psychologist Henri Tajfel and his colleagues conducted minimal-group studies, which showed that people identified as members of a group simply by being categorised into that group (Ellemers 2019). Tajfel and Turner (1979) outlined a theory (social identity theory) to observe intergroup behaviour and intergroup conflict, specifically applying the theory to individual prejudice and discrimination through interpersonal behaviour. Their study elucidated that intergroup conflict or competition facilitated, for instance, greater intragroup morale, which is linked to interpersonal behaviour (Tajfel and Turner 1979).

The 1970 minimal-group studies allowed for the development of social identity theory. Following Tajfel and Turner (1979), scholars have applied the theory across various disciplines. Leaper (2011) stated that the theory addressed the ways in which social identities affected individuals' attitudes and behaviours regarding their ingroup and outgroup membership. The theory has three main dimensions, which include social categorisation, social identification and social comparison (Tajfel and Turner 1979). Social categorisation allows individuals to categorise objects to understand their meaning and identify them, helping understand the context and social environment (McLeod 2019; Tajfel and Turner 1979). Social identification occurs when individuals adopt the identity of the group that they have categorised themselves as belonging to, meaning that they conform to the norms of that group and attach emotional significance to their identification with that group (McLeod 2019). This provides a "system of orientation for self-reference" whereby "they create and define the individual's place in society" (Tajfel and Turner 1979, p. 40), as participants did in this study. Social comparison refers to categorising and identifying with a group and comparing one's group with other groups (McLeod 2019). Tajfel and Turner (1979) described social comparison as relational and comparative, defining individuals as 'better' or 'worse' than members of other groups. These dimensions strongly link to social identity and can be applied to understand participants' perceptions of their identities.

Social identity refers to people's self-concepts based on their membership in social groups and how they categorise themselves in social groups (Leaper 2011; Tajfel and Turner 1979). Jenkins (2014) argued that the 'social' part of 'social identity' was redundant and described (social) identity as how individuals identify themselves, depending on the context of the situation. It involves interaction through communication and negotiation (of one's identity). This study found that DNA test results affected participants' social or group identities, making social identity theory valuable in this research and reflecting the varied perspectives that participants held.

5. Methodology

A qualitative approach was used in this study to contextualise participants' interviews and their perceptions of their identities. Vaismoradi and Snelgrove (2019) described the aim of qualitative research to help provide "cultural and contextual description and interpretation of [a] social phenomenon" (p. 1). According to Jamshed (2014), interviewing and observations are the most common qualitative methods of data collection. Such interviews can be very open, using narrative interviewing, flexibly structured interviews or focus groups (Scholl 2015). Interviews, as a qualitative method (Cavana et al. 2001), were selected to give further insight into participants' perceptions.

5.1. Interviews

Interviews were semi-structured and in-depth, allowing for mutability in participants' answers. Part of this process included guiding the participant with open-ended questions and ascertaining when to ask further questions for deeper understanding and context of the participant's narrative (Galletta 2013). Jamshed (2014) described semi-structured interviews as having a partially structured guide of questions that the interviewer would explore during the interview, and in order to optimise time, these guides allow for focused and comprehensive answers from interviewees. Schlütz and Möhring (2015) described in-depth interviews as open-ended interviews, where these types of interviews "reconstruct social events as first-hand experience via storytelling" (p. 302). In the case of the current research, it was important to keep these points in mind and to rearrange questions during the interviews, enabling an interactive approach, allowing for openness of communication and providing opportunities for participants to express their perspectives of how DNA test results affected their identities while also conforming to how Galletta (2013) and Cavana et al. (2001) emphasised the idea of the 'researcher as an instrument', where one can prompt participants, rephrase questions and make changes depending on the interview situation.

Cavana et al. (2001) described face-to-face interviews as information gathering where the interviewer and interviewee meet in person. Interviews were devised to be face to face and were conducted in person where possible as part of the data collection, but with the emergence of easily accessible digital applications, such as Skype, Zoom, Facebook and Microsoft Teams, face-to-face connection could be made visually without meeting in person. Having this face-to-face communication was important in fostering relationships, having good communication, giving opportunities for information and questions to be revisited and helping facilitate more open discussion. Participants who were not interviewed in person were interviewed through their preferred video calling channel (usually Facebook Messenger or Skype).

The indicative interview questions are available in Appendix A. Further information about the type of interview (in-person or video call), how long each interview was and the location of each participant during the time of the interview is available in the link to the study mentioned in the 'Data Availability Statement'.

5.2. Sampling

In order to find participants, purposive sampling and iterations of snowball sampling were used to connect with possible networks and find further networks where participants would likely fit the inclusion criteria (such as participants completing a DNA test and receiving their results, or would be receiving their results before the interview). For 'purposive' sampling, the size of the sample depended on the number of factors relevant to the study's purpose (Merriam and Tisdell 2016). The researcher initially posted publicly on their Facebook and LinkedIn pages to reach potential participants and allow for sharing across further networks through word of mouth. This is similar to how Audemard (2020) described snowball sampling as involving a first sample of informants who then refer and help recruit participants. Snowball sampling focuses on using two populations: the individual and their relationships (Coleman 1958; Audemard 2020).

To gain a wider reach, multiple groups associated with genealogy were contacted, as genealogists frequently perform DNA tests to assist their research. These included the 'New Zealand Society of Genealogists (NZSG)' and two Facebook pages: 'Genealogy New Zealand and Beyond' and 'Using DNA for Genealogy—Australia & NZ'. Contacting these networks was similar to applying the snowball sampling method, as it utilised the networks of a designated person branching out (Audemard 2020). As a result, a total of sixteen participants were found for the interviews.

5.3. Thematic Analysis

A thematic analysis was used to analyse the interview data. Thematic analysis focuses on themes and patterns in the data, "identifying, analysing, and reporting patterns (themes) within data" (Braun and Clarke 2006, p. 83). Key phases include (1) familiarisation with the data, (2) generating initial codes, (3) searching for themes, (4) reviewing themes, (5) defining and naming themes and (6) producing the report (Braun and Clarke 2006). In order to become more familiar with the data, the audio collected through the interviews was roughly transcribed using otter.ai (an artificial intelligence program that transcribes audio into text) to provide a basic verbatim transcript, along with the use of the video interviews for reference to provide an overall understanding and context.

The researcher manually revised the transcription to remove inaccuracies, and then used verbatim transcripts in conjunction with handwritten notes to identify common semantic features relating to the research question of 'how do DNA test results affect individuals' perceptions of their identity/identities?'. This allowed for the generation of the initial codes by using semantic coding from the transcripts and thereby going through the second phase of Braun and Clarke's (2006) thematic analysis. Vaismoradi and Snelgrove (2019) described the generation of initial codes as being done by highlighting the main ideas as codes in relation to the topic. Braun and Clarke (2019) explained the differentiation between a code and a theme as the code being more specific, capturing a single idea within a segment of data, which can be a 'building block' to create a theme. This type of thematic analysis is commonly a recursive process that moves between each of the six phases; the analytic approach may blend some of these phases together (Braun and Clarke n.d.), as is evident in the latter three phases. A theme "captures a common, recurring pattern across a dataset, clustered around a central organising concept" (Braun and Clarke 2019, p. 2). Further to the semantic content of the data collected, a latent approach delved into the understanding of the implicit and underlying meaning, looking at the form and meaning of the data (Braun and Clarke 2006; Lainson et al. 2019). For the purpose of this research, themes were created through a semantic approach. Braun and Clarke (2006) explained this as a process where the researcher identifies themes by looking at the explicit or surface meaning of what the participant has said or written—in this case, what the participants said and what was transcribed. After the development and finalisation of themes, the findings and discussion were produced, thereby enacting the sixth and final phase of the thematic analysis.

6. Findings and Discussion

The finalised themes from the full study's thematic analysis included: family belonging, genealogy and ancestry, genetic family connection, family stories, place belonging, group belonging, national pride, unexpected information, cultural affinity and seeking answers. The full findings from the analysis are available through the link in the 'Data Availability Statement'. Although there are elements of overlap between themes, there are distinct aspects to each theme presented in Table 1. This article focuses on family belonging, unexpected information and seeking answers, which are elaborated in the following discussion sections: 'DNA test results reinforcing or contradicting identity claims', 'seeking answers to find family identities' and 'unexpected information prompting identity adaptation'. Moreover, participants will be referred to by their initials throughout the discussion (for instance, CR).

Table 1. Theme summary.

Theme	Description
Family Belonging	Participants' feelings of belonging to a family or their feelings of not belonging to their perceived family group and their desire to be a part of their family[ies].
Seeking Answers	After receiving unexpected information, participants wanted answers and the truth about family members, specifically their close family relationships of their parent(s) and/or grandparent(s).
Unexpected Information	Participants finding unexpected information as a result of their DNA tests, creating further interest in seeking answers.

6.1. DNA Test Results Reinforcing or Contradicting Family Identity Claims

Discrepancies in the DNA test results noted by participants prompted re-negotiation of identities and affected their feelings of belonging to their perceived social groups, especially their family and biological groups. For some, the results reinforced their identity claims, whereas those with results contradicting these claims had their identities strongly affected, highlighting how socially constructed groups fostered their belonging and feelings of being connected.

Shim et al. (2018) stated that "[i]deas about oneself in relation to others, perceptions of how others see oneself, one's treatment by others, are all the product of processual, cumulative, lived and indelibly social experiences" (p. 44). Although Shim et al. (2018) focused on racial identity, the notion of having lived experiences constructing one's identity is relevant and applicable to other identities. Participants in this study mentioned communication being used to foster their group belonging, but overwhelmingly mentioned their feelings of belonging to a family group. Family is a socially constructed group, and the feeling of belonging to this group was evident in participants' narratives about their DNA results. Because of their DNA test results, the participants exhibited a change in perception of their family identity or, in some cases, adopted multiple family identities when their DNA results were different from their family identity claims. For instance, when KB learned that her biological father was someone different, she consequently met her biological father and his two children, along with another half-sister from another family (fathered by her biological father), as well as her grandmother and cousins. She also expressed occasionally feeling a lack of belonging in the family she was raised in, feeling left out of gatherings, especially during a family event in which her grandmother commented that her father was the local pub owner, which "scared" her.

'Family' is defined by LEXICO (n.d.) as meaning "[a] group of one or more parents and their children living together as a unit" (para. 1) or "[a]ll the descendants of a common ancestor" (para. 4). More recently, a further definition was added: "a group of related things" (LEXICO n.d., para. 7); this encapsulates the changing notions of family. Participants used these three definitions interchangeably when talking about their immediate family and extended family through DNA matches, as well as their biological family and the family in which they were raised.

A lack of belonging to their 'family' was usually due to a change in their perceived identity through unexpected DNA test results. In many cases, the unexpected results prompted an identity crisis (the disturbances that disrupt the self) and affected their ego identity (the psychic structure fundamental to psychological equilibrium) (Coulmas 2019; Fearon 1999; Harvard University n.d.; Izenberg 2016). Although these disruptions were not age-specific, they disturbed the sense of self and contributed to who they believed themselves to be, thereby affecting their wider relationships.

For example, CR felt that she had a significant change in her perceived identity after her DNA test did not show DNA matches with her expected biological grandfather. She stated that a quarter of who she thought she was now unknown. By exploring the possibilities of the unknown quarter, she was re-evaluating her family relationships and who she was as a member of this familial group. Her actions displayed a disruption in her sense of self and expressed elements of social identity theory. As described prior, social identity theory refers to the interplay between personal and social identities and attempts to specify and predict the circumstances of how one perceives oneself as an individual or as a group member (Ellemers 2019; McLeod 2019). Tajfel and Turner (1979) described the feeling of membership as 'social identity', whereby one's self-image is derived from the social categories to which individuals perceive themselves as belonging. This can be seen through CR's feeling of having a significant change in her perceived identity and her questioning of what her biological family would be like, even though she loved the family that raised her. This reinforces the idea that identities are most important when individuals feel that they have strong emotional ties to a group and have membership with that group, thereby reinforcing their self-esteem, which sustains their social identity (Leaper 2011). Disruption, therefore, caused participants such as CR to re-evaluate these emotional ties and the effects on their identities.

One of the three dimensions of social identity, social categorisation, was evident in the way that CR categorised her family relationships when referring to her "biological family" and the family that raised her and, therefore, categorising these relationships to understand her context and social environment (McLeod 2019; Tajfel and Turner 1979).

CR had revisited her DNA results and looked at the names only to find that her grandfather was not her biological grandfather; she mentioned, "It's impacted me immensely because a quarter of who I thought I was I'm not and it's a very odd sensation; it's an odd feeling in not knowing now". She added that she was surprised how much it impacted who she believed herself to be, as her whole family line from Manchester, England was no longer what she thought it was. By acknowledging these separate categories, CR became associated with two family identities, which shows how DNA test results can solidify or separate familial identities.

CR further questioned what her biological family would be like, comparing herself to the two families and looking for potential similarities. This process has some semblance with social comparison, another dimension of social identity theory. This dimension refers to categorising and identifying with a group and comparing that group to other groups, which are usually relational (McLeod 2019; Tajfel and Turner 1979). In this case, CR described her membership in her biological family and the family that raised her as having membership in two different groups—one in a biological sense, and the other in what she had believed to be her family identity. Effectively, she socially compared herself, redefined her group belonging and associated herself with two distinct family groups.

CR also used the term "love" in aligning herself with the family that she was raised in and described feeling a sense of belonging, which was much like how NH described feelings of belonging when asking her grandmother questions about their relations and how RG talked about one of her favourite stories because it showed their family having fun together:

> My uncles would play the fiddle, and all those little things, I don't even know the proper names of everything, and we would have things like barn dances. So that was who I was growing up.

These participants associated themselves with a family group and their positive shared experiences, describing the relational element that made them feel included and part of the family. This is similar to achieving satisfactory group identification, which can be described as a sense of belonging formed by group identities that are relational and that include peers and exclude others (Coulmas 2019). Walker (2015) also described love as having a crucial role in "a sense of safety and belonging" (p. 102). Although Walker's (2015) research focused on child adoptees, the feeling of belonging to a family is relevant to these participants' perceptions of their identity and reflects that belonging is often intertwined with strong emotions—in this case, positive emotions.

It was evident that relationships were reflected on by these participants, reinforcing the idea that families have their own group boundaries and identities. Soliz and Harwood (2006) described families as having 'intergroup' and 'intragroup' relationships, where family members share an inherent ingroup for all members, but also have individual identities that show intragroup boundaries within the family. Thus, participants' positive emotive affiliations reinforced their family belonging and the relationships within each family group, even when familial identities were separated. The participants' narratives demonstrated that they looked for inclusion in order to retain separate identities or placed more value on their biological identity. When this inclusion was disrupted, as was the case for certain participants, their sense of identity was affected.

For example, BD had identified with the English side of her family until she was nursing someone with haemophilia and her mother was prompted to tell her that she [the mother] was adopted. BD recounted that she was "horrified because I love my grandparents. That to me, it was huge. Suddenly they weren't my grandparents". This demonstrates another dimension in social identity theory, namely, social identification. Social identification occurs when individuals adopt the identity of the group they have categorised themselves as belonging to by conforming to the norms of the group and attaching an emotional significance to their identification with the group (McLeod 2019). This dimension also provides a reference for an individual to create and define their place in society (Tajfel and Turner 1979). Therefore, with participants attaching emotional significance to their identification with their social (and familial) identities, unexpected information as in the cases of CR and BD can change perspectives and the ways that they identify themselves. This may lead to feelings of exclusion from their perceived family groups.

Although DNA test results can cause this drastic change in social and familial identities, DNA matches also allowed these participants to try to get in contact with those who could help them find more information, thus allowing for inclusion in another group and a sense of belonging within their 'current' family. These matches can mitigate the effect of an identity crisis by providing answers and support. CR and BD expressed "love" for their family members, suggesting strong emotional attachment, and thus, it was a greater shock to find out their biological identities did not match their perceived family identities. However, JG also experienced misalignment of these identities, but said that the results and new information about her biological father not being who she thought did not affect her. JG said she felt "very fortunate" because "they were both so much older". Her mother was thirty-seven, and both her biological father (the local gynaecologist) and the father who she had been raised by were both in their fifties when she was born. From this, she said:

> I didn't do a lot with my father, with my legal father. I could count on one hand the number of times we actually went and did something together, just us together because he was so much older.

She was aware that her mother wanted a child and was struggling to have one, so she believed that her biological father was a "pioneer in gynaecology and women's reproductive systems. And [it was] very well known that the women of Wagga thought he was just wonderful. I don't know what that might mean." JG said that she loved the family she grew up in and was still happy to be in contact with them, showing that the participants articulated different impacts on their identities. A positive emotional significance can reinforce family belonging by fostering relationships and strengthening family identities. However, it can also cause re-evaluation of this identity and individuals' belonging within the group.

It can be argued that the notions of family are continually shifting and cannot be clearly outlined, as is evident with the addition of the definition of 'family' to LEXICO's (n.d.) dictionary. This is similar to Isensee's (2015) claim that notions of family have come under more scrutiny in recent years, as family was usually defined within the nuclear family dynamic (consisting of married parents and their biological or adopted children). However, family is socially constructed and the participants had varied perceptions on what constituted their families.

LEXICO's (n.d.) additional definition of family that describes a 'group of related things' shows that notions of family are changing, allowing for more variance than the original definition of purely being part of a 'family unit' or 'descendants of a common ancestor'. It also demonstrates that definitions of family may be different from one's familial or biological identities. In some cases, such as those of KB, CR, BD and JG, participants may have lived in a family unit when DNA test results revealed that the family they thought they belonged to was not fully biologically connected. Nevertheless, they still associated this unit with one of their family identities. This reframing of their family identities conforms with claims from authors such as Stallard and Groot (2020, p. 289), who stated that DNA test results:

> can be disruptive, and often individuals are resistant to redefining the family group. In the case of special groups like adoptees, those with unknown parents, those with half-sibs and stepsiblings, new information can shatter the model of family identity that had been built up for many years.

With DNA test results having an immediate effect on test takers' lives, they have increased the likelihood of disrupting their senses of self and group belonging whilst forming connections to other identities and shared experiences. This is in line with some concluding remarks made by Shim et al. (2018), where they found that "participants' racial identities emanated from their cumulative, personal, familial and social life experiences—and therefore as discrete from information they received from a singular source (their genetics) at one point in time" (p. 58).

6.2. Seeking Answers to Find Family Identities

For most participants with substantial changes in their perceived family identities (unexpected results about parents or grandparents), there was a significant change in the sense of self and a desire to seek the truth. They sought answers about their family members to help them understand who they were and where they belonged. In other words, there was a change in their familial and personal identities. For example, JG had unexpected results about her biological father, but she was able to use her DNA matches to find some of the answers to her questions. Comparatively, CR, KB and BD all wanted further answers and explanations for why their DNA tests revealed unexpected results. Their families had not discussed the possibilities or were not able to give clarity about why there were unexpected results.

When CR found out that her biological grandfather was not who she thought, she reflected on "this whole family I never got to know and I still don't know. How do I build that connection now?". KB, who found that her biological father was not who she thought and who has since reconnected with biological family members, said for a long time that she felt "robbed" of what could have been her life if she had been raised with her biological sisters or father. Connections to people were clearly important to her sense of self. She did, however, say that she had worked through it and, in the end, felt that she "had the best possible life" and that she was "grateful" for the life she had. These emotive phrases correspond with affective understanding in looking at belonging in the context of others, which is in line with Wood's and Black's (2016; as cited in Turner 2019) research.

This shows the affective understanding and importance of relationships to one's identities and, importantly, how disruption affects a person's sense of identity. The connection through family that CR mentioned and the participants' use of affective and emotive language when describing their family connections reaffirm that family is one of the most fundamental and important social groups for individuals (Soliz and Harwood 2006; Colaner et al. 2018).

For some, family may be the most important social group, but other social groups can also hold strong importance. Belonging is important for participants' identities (Wood and Black 2016; as cited in Turner 2019). Thus, feeling belonging through relationships seems to be a fundamental aspect that resonates with various social groups, including family. The degree to which people perceive themselves as part of an in-group (such as a family) and have shared relational culture is important, thereby marking their identification with the group (Soliz and Rittenour 2012; as cited in Colaner et al. 2018). As the intergroup research of Soliz et al. (2009) revealed, there were benefits to individuals forming a cohesive shared family identity because it facilitated a shared belonging within a family.

Participants' questioning of their shared family identities resulted in more questions about themselves as individuals, as was the case with CR and BD. Without answers to their questions, participants used further emotive words to describe their feelings of emptiness. CR felt "vacant" and said, "we [she and her mother] feel like we're in limbo". KB and BD also expressed a shift in their perception of who they thought they were and wanted answers. BD articulated a similar sense of emptiness to that of CR, but was able to find partial answers, as she had met her biological grandfather's family, although she was still searching for her biological grandmother's identity. These participants wanted truthful answers in order to understand their own place within the family and their individual identities to find out where they came from, as well as their relationships and connections with their parents/grandparents. This was much like how Stallard and Groot (2020) described how those who were searching for parents or grandparents (such as BD, who was looking for her birth grandfather) used DNA tests to "discover results that could significantly reconfigure their familial identity and relationships" (p. 287). These findings highlighted the importance of familial relationships in determining one's belonging and the role of DNA testing in helping achieve this.

Having strong relationships with parents and grandparents resembles Soliz and Harwood's (2006) study on shared family identity. Their study focused on the grandparent–grandchild relationship, showing that "personal communication emerged as a strong influential factor in perceptions of shared family identity across all grandparents" (p. 100). Therefore, a strong relationship with one's grandparents and, in this case, one's parents increases the likelihood that those who have undergone a substantial shift will have to realign their perceived shared family identities.

Again, these findings reinforce the importance of relationships and feelings (affective understanding) as part of belonging (Wood and Black 2016; as cited in Turner 2019).

There are similarities with how Nash (2004) described the increased popularisation of genetic testing as creating 'genetic kinship' and how this knowledge creates "new definitions of gender, 'race' and relative that reinforce, reshape or challenge existing notions of collective identity and personhood" (p. 4). Since then, the latter was most important in relation to participants who were seeking answers about their family identities. Having 'genetic kinship' allows for a sense of group belonging, and similarities in DNA create a sense of potential connection and possible relationships.

6.3. Unexpected Information Prompting Identity Adaptation

In this study, the majority of the participants' stories showed that DNA tests affected individuals' perceptions of their identities. Unexpected information as a result of these tests was undoubtedly one of the most prominent factors.

However, such discoveries through DNA testing also prompted interest in exploring possible identities. CH wanted to find her Korean origins because no one in her family was aware of the connection. Similarly, NH said that she had very unexpected results, with her ethnicity estimates showing 20% Italian. She assumed this could be connected to her maternal grandfather's side, about whom she did not know much, but she was surprised that her two brothers did not have any Italian in their estimates. AV was also surprised by her "Baltic blood", showing "Lithuania and Latvia" in her ethnicity estimates. She had expected Russia and maybe some estimates from Ukraine, Poland or Slovakia, but hoped for something such as Brazil. CH, NH and AV alluded to their biogeographic ancestry and biological identity making them feel connected to an area, with their tests prompting interest in learning more about these areas and their relationships with their family identities. Instead of changing their perceived identities, they showed an interest in broadening their understanding of their own identities.

DJ's Y-DNA test results allowed him to find a Scottish connection with his paternal haplogroup, which had "never entered into the conversation", thus forming his Scottish pride, as well as a feeling of belonging to a new clan and being biologically connected to family through one lineage. Other family relationships were also fostered through unexpected information. CR revisited her DNA test results and was surprised about the impact that this had on her, as she questioned her personal and family identities.

As mentioned earlier in this article, participants' use of emotive phrases reflected their affective understanding of exploring their belonging (Wood and Black 2016; as cited in Turner 2019). Participants expressed that the unexpected results created varied emotions, with most being "surprised" by their ethnicity estimates. Others who had to renavigate their family relationships seemed to have a more substantial emotional disturbance in their senses of self, as evidenced by CR saying that it impacted her "immensely because a quarter of who I thought I was I'm not". Disruption in her identity was evident with her unexpected results, showing that there was an emotional fallout when receiving confusing or life-changing test results, where "[i]dentities that have been cherished by families for generations can be dismantled overnight" (Lawton 2018, para. 6). As more people take DNA tests, the possibility of identity disruption is becoming increasingly likely.

Despite being an adult, CR also expressed genealogical bewilderment, which can be described as "potential identity problems that can be experienced by a child who has been separated from her birth parents" (Walker 2015, p. 93). Whilst she was not separated from her birth parents, she exhibited the overall meaning of the term, where genealogical bewilderment may include questions about who one is and where one belongs (Walker 2015).

KB also experienced genealogical bewilderment. She connected with new biological family members after coming to terms with her unexpected results, finding another half-sister on her paternal side although her biological half-sister's parents denied the validity of the test. Her experience conformed to Stallard and Groot's (2020) assertion that those receiving DNA test results can be resistant to having to redefine their family groups. Although KB redefined her new belonging within another family (her biological family) and attempted to help her newfound biological half-sister renavigate identities, her half-sister's family did not. In terms of relationships, feeling and space (Wood and Black 2016;

as cited in Turner 2019), KB renegotiated her identity, helping another biologically related individual in the same situation. This reinforced the potential of DNA complicating the notion of family while also broadening possibilities (Stallard and Groot 2020).

Likewise, JG found a DNA match that was likely to be her half great niece, which led her to find out that there was a problem with her birth father (as she did not have any siblings). She described this as "completely and absolutely, and utterly unexpected". When she did further research, she found that her biological father was the local gynaecologist in the town in which she was born, and so believed that her birth may have been the result of him being a "pioneer in gynaecology" (suggesting that he may have had an understanding about practices such as artificial insemination). However, JG seemingly focused her realignment of her identity with her autobiographical completeness, trying to understand her unexpected results and how they shaped her understanding of self, whereas CR and KB had to re-evaluate their family identities and new relationships, rather than solely focusing on their autobiographical completeness. Autobiographical and genealogical connectedness were mentioned by Walker (2015), who wrote about children's psychological development, where one uses elements of connectedness to create a sense of belonging, a coherent sense of self and a clear identity.

7. Conclusions

This study highlighted some of the effects of DNA test results on participants' identities. Belonging to a family group and feeling 'connected' were key elements in participants' sense of self and transcended multiple identities.

With genetic testing revealing DNA matches that increase as more biological relatives take the test, people who test in the future may also have unexpected results, forcing them to renegotiate their family identities. This may be beneficial to some testers, but could equally change their perspectives. These test results may increase their feeling of inclusion in a (family) group and, therefore, their feeling of a sense of belonging to their family, or they may feel excluded and look for answers. They may even feel a certain degree of belonging to both their biological relatives and the family that they grew up with, thus changing their perception of their family[ies] and what constitutes their family identity[ies]. Feelings of belonging with multiple group identities elucidate the changing notions of family.

'Family' increasingly encapsulates multiple identities and will continue to be challenged and refined as more DNA tests are taken and further developments are made with genetic technology. Even though aspects of family may be biologically shaped, the lived-in environments are equally important in determining one's feeling of belonging and connection. Relationships were evidently important, with biological connections reaffirming participants' identities and discrepancies altering their relationships and perspectives of personal and group identity.

Recommendations for future research include looking at how DNA test results affect further disruptions in identity, including cases such as individuals who were separated from families through wars and conflicts, as well as adoptions. Looking at their perceived identities and feelings of belonging would be a useful addition for understanding the importance of lived-in and biological family and relationship dynamics.

Overall, participants' associations were positive and inquisitive. Despite some unexpected results, they all acknowledged new or different aspects of their identities, prompting some identity re-alignment. In some cases, unexpected results were not as significant to their senses of self or group belonging because they attached more importance to other identities. Individuals hold multiple identities, each with their own importance, and the participants were ultimately looking for some semblance of belonging or connection.

Funding: This research received no external funding.

Institutional Review Board Statement: This research obtained ethics approval 19/301 from the Auckland University of Technology Ethics Committee on 10 September 2019.

Informed Consent Statement: Informed consent was obtained from all subjects involved in the study.

Data Availability Statement: Full findings, appendices of interviews, questions and participant summaries are available at https://openrepository.aut.ac.nz/handle/10292/14111 (accessed on 2 December 2021).

Acknowledgments: A substantial thank you to all the participants who shared their stories as part of this research. Also, a thank you to the New Zealand Society of Genealogists (NZSG), and the two Facebook groups 'Genealogy New Zealand and Beyond' and 'Using DNA for Genealogy—Australia & NZ', who helped facilitate the finding of participants.

Conflicts of Interest: The author declares no conflict of interest.

Appendix A

Indicative questions used in the interviews:

- Can you tell me a story that resonates with your identity?
- How did your DNA test results affect this?
- Do you feel like it impacted your identity in any other ways?
- Did you find out anything about yourself that was unexpected?
- What test did you take and what did you initially expect?
- Has the test changed your perspective at all?
- Since you got the DNA test results, do you have a recent story that resonates with your identity (whether it's the same or changed)?
- Will you be taking any further steps to get more information since the DNA test or is this a one-off?
- Is there anything you'd like to add?

References

23andMe, Inc. n.d. 23andMe Homepage. Available online: https://www.23andme.com/ (accessed on 22 November 2021).
AncestryDNA. n.d. Uncover More of Your Story. Available online: https://www.ancestry.com.au/dna/ (accessed on 20 November 2021).
Anderson, Alyssa. 2021. What Are Autosomal DNA Tests? WebMD. Available online: https://www.webmd.com/a-to-z-guides/what-are-autosomal-dna-tests (accessed on 9 November 2021).
Anzilotti, Amy W. 2021. Genetic Testing. Kids Health from Nemours. Available online: https://kidshealth.org/en/parents/genetics.html (accessed on 6 February 2022).
Audemard, Julien. 2020. Objectifying contextual effects. The use of snowball sampling in political sociology. *BMS: Bulletin de Methodologie Sociologigue* 145: 30–60. [CrossRef]
Bernath, Viviana. 2015. *Social Identity and Biological Identity*. Translated by Jane Ramirez. Ann Arbor: U-M Center for Latin American and Caribbean Studies, vol. 3, pp. 35–86. [CrossRef]
Best Tests. 2014. Genetic Health Services New Zealand (GHSNZ): What You Need to Know. BPAC Medicine. Available online: https://bpac.org.nz/BT/2014/November/docs/BT25-ghsnz.pdf (accessed on 25 November 2021).
Braun, Virginia, and Victoria Clarke. 2006. Using thematic analysis in psychology. *Qualitative Research in Psychology* 3: 77–101. [CrossRef]
Braun, Virginia, and Victoria Clarke. 2019. Answers to Frequently Asked Questions about Thematic Analysis. The University of Auckland. Available online: https://cdn.auckland.ac.nz/assets/psych/about/our-research/documents/Answers%20to%20frequently%20asked%20questions%20about%20thematic%20analysis%20April%202019.pdf (accessed on 8 October 2019).
Braun, Virginia, and Victoria Clarke. n.d. Thematic Analysisa Reflexive Approach. The University of Auckland. Available online: https://www.psych.auckland.ac.nz/en/about/thematic-analysis.html (accessed on 8 October 2019).
Cavana, Robert Y., Brian L. Delahaye, and Uma Sekaran. 2001. *Applied Business Research: Qualitative and Quantitative Methods*. Hoboken: Wiley.
Colaner, Colleen Warne, Haley Kranstuber Horstman, and Christine E. Rittenour. 2018. Negotiating adoptive and birth shared family identity: A social identity complexity approach. *Western Journal of Communication* 82: 393–415. [CrossRef]
Coleman, James S. 1958. Relational Analysis: The Study of Social Organizations with Survey Methods. *Human Organization* 17: 28–36. Available online: https://www.jstor.org/stable/44124097 (accessed on 5 October 2019). [CrossRef]
Coulmas, Florian. 2019. *Identity: A Very Short Introduction*. Oxford: Oxford University Press. [CrossRef]

Darroch, Fiona, and Ian Smith. 2021. Establishing Identity: How Direct-To-Consumer Genetic Testing Challenges the Assumption of Donor Anonymity. *Family Court Review* 59: 103–20. Available online: https://onlinelibrary.wiley.com/doi/epdf/10.1111/fcre.12553 (accessed on 5 February 2022). [CrossRef]

Dooney, Laura. 2017. Native Affairs Reveal DNA Test of Full-Blooded Māori Woman. Stuff NZ. Available online: https://www.stuff.co.nz/national/91480531/native-affairs-reveal-dna-test-of-fullblooded-maori-woman?rm=m (accessed on 12 April 2017).

Ellemers, Naomi. 2019. Social Identity Theory. In *Encyclopaedia Britannica*. Available online: https://www.britannica.com/topic/social-identity-theory (accessed on 4 January 2019).

Elliott, Carl, and Paul Brodwin. 2002. Identity and genetic ancestry tracing. *BMJ* 325: 1469–71. [CrossRef] [PubMed]

Fearon, James D. 1999. *What Is Identity (as We Now Use the Word)?* Stanford: Stanford University. Available online: https://web.stanford.edu/group/fearon-research/cgi-bin/wordpress/wp-content/uploads/2013/10/What-is-Identity-as-we-now-use-the-word-.pdf (accessed on 20 October 2019).

Galletta, Anne. 2013. *Mastering the Semi-Structured Interview and beyond: From Research Design to Analysis and Publication*. New York: New York University Press. Available online: https://www.jstor.org/stable/j.ctt9qgh5x (accessed on 10 October 2019).

Gene by Gene, Ltd. n.d. FamilyTreeDNA Homepage. Available online: https://www.familytreedna.com/ (accessed on 22 November 2021).

Harvard University. n.d. Erik Erikson (1902–1994). Available online: https://psychology.fas.harvard.edu/people/erik-erikson (accessed on 7 April 2020).

Isensee, Reinhard. 2015. Introduction. In *Family and Kinship in the United States, Cultural Perspectives on Familial Belonging*, 1st ed. Edited by Karolina Golimowska, Reinhard Isensee and David Rose. Location: Peter Lang Edition, pp. 7–14.

Izenberg, Gerald. 2016. *Identity, the Necessity of a Modern Idea*. Pennsylvania: University of Pennsylvania Press.

Jamshed, Shazia. 2014. Qualitative research method-interviewing and observation. *Journal of Basic and Clinical Pharmacy* 5: 87–88. [CrossRef]

Jenkins, Richard. 2014. *Social Identity*, 4th ed. London: Routledge.

Jhamb, Kamna. 2021. Direct to Consumer Testing Industry Global Markets (HLC269A). BCC Publishing. Available online: https://www.bccresearch.com/market-research/healthcare/direct-to-consumer-testing-market.html (accessed on 16 November 2021).

King, Turi E., and Mark A. Jobling. 2009. What's in a name? Y chromosomes, surnames and the genetic genealogy revolution. *Trends in Genetics* 25: 351–60. [CrossRef]

Lainson, Kristina, Virginia Braun, and Victoria Clarke. 2019. Being Both Narrative Practitioner and Academic Researcher: A Reflection on What Thematic Analysis Has to Offer Narratively Informed Research. *International Journal of Narrative Therapy and Community Work* 4: 86–98. Available online: https://uwe-repository.worktribe.com/output/4820836/being-both-narrative-practitioner-and-academic-researcher-a-reflection-on-what-thematic-analysis-has-to-offer-narratively-informed-research (accessed on 15 October 2019).

Lawton, Bessie, and Anita Foeman. 2017. Shifting Winds: Using Ancestry DNA to Explore Multiracial Individual's Patterns of Articulating Racial Identity. *Identity* 17: 69–83. [CrossRef]

Lawton, Georgina. 2018. It Made Me Question My Ancestry': Does DNA Home Testing Really Understand Race? *The Guardian*. August 11. Available online: https://www.theguardian.com/lifeandstyle/2018/aug/11/question-ancestry-does-dna-testing-really-understand-race (accessed on 29 September 2019).

Leaper, Campbell. 2011. More similarities than differences in contemporary theories of social development? *Advances in Child Development and Behaviour* 40: 337–78. [CrossRef]

LEXICO. n.d. Definition of Family in English: Family. In *Oxford English and Spanish Dictionary, Thesaurus, and Spanish to English Translator*. Available online: https://www.lexico.com/en/definition/family (accessed on 29 November 2021).

LivingDNA Ltd. n.d. The Most Advanced DNA Test to Discover Your Ancestry. Available online: https://livingdna.com/nz/kit/ancestry-dna-test (accessed on 22 November 2021).

McLeod, Saul A. 2019. Social Identity Theory. *Simply Psychology*. October 24. Available online: https://www.simplypsychology.org/social-identity-theory.html (accessed on 10 February 2020).

Medline Plus. 2020. What Is Genetic Ancestry Testing? In *NIH U.S. National Library of Medicine*; September 21. Available online: https://ghr.nlm.nih.gov/primer/dtcgenetictesting/ancestrytesting (accessed on 20 September 2020).

Merriam, Sharan B., and Elizabeth J. Tisdell. 2016. *Qualitative Research: A Guide to Design and Implementation*, 4th ed. San Francisco: Jossey-Bass.

MyHeritage. n.d. Discover Your Family Story. Available online: https://www.myheritage.com/dna (accessed on 22 November 2021).

Nash, Catherine. 2004. Genetic kinship. *Cultural Studies* 18: 1–33. [CrossRef]

National Human Genome Research Institute. 2018. Human Genome Project Timeline of Events. Available online: https://www.genome.gov/human-genome-project/Timeline-of-Events (accessed on 12 April 2020).

Puig, Pere, Anna Barceló, Roger Lahoz, Àngels Niubó, Jimi Jiménez, Montserrat Soler-López, Michael J. Donovan, Joaquima Navarro, Jordi Camps, Montserrat Garcia-Caldés, and et al. 2019. Genetic identification of a war-evacuated child in search of his own identity for more than seventy years. *Forensic Science International* 298: 312–15. [CrossRef] [PubMed]

Schlütz, Daniela, and Wiebke Möhring. 2015. Interview, Qualitative. In *The Concise Encyclopaedia of Communication*, 1st ed. Edited by Wolfgang Donsbach. Hoboken: John Wiley & Sons, Inc., pp. 301–2.

Schneider, Peter M., Barbara Prainsack, and Manfred Kayser. 2019. The use of forensic DNA phenotyping in predicting appearance and biogeographic ancestry. *Deutsches Aerzteblatt International* 116: 873–80. [CrossRef]

Scholl, Armin. 2015. Qualitative Methodology. In *The Concise Encyclopaedia of Communication*, 1st ed. Edited by Wolfgang Donsbach. Hoboken: John Wiley & Sons, Inc., pp. 510–12.

Shim, Janet K., Sonia Rab Alam, and Bradley E. Aouizerat. 2018. Knowing something verses feeling different: The effects and non-effects of genetic ancestry on racial identity. *New Genetics and Society* 37: 44–66. [CrossRef]

Soliz, Jordan, Allison R. Thorson, and Christine E. Rittenour. 2009. Communicative correlates of satisfaction, family identity, and group salience in multiracial/ethnic families. *Journal of Marriage and Family* 71: 819–32. [CrossRef]

Soliz, Jordan, and Christine E. Rittenour. 2012. Family as an intergroup arena. In *The Handbook of Intergroup Communication*. Edited by Howard Giles. London: Routledge, pp. 331–43.

Soliz, Jordan, and Jake Harwood. 2006. Shared family identity, age salience, and intergroup contact: Investigation of the grandparent-grandchild relationship. *Communication Monographs* 73: 87–107. [CrossRef]

Stallard, Matthew, and Jerome de Groot. 2020. "Thing are coming out that are questionable, we never knew about": DNA and the new family history. *Journal of Family History* 45: 274–94. [CrossRef]

Strand, Daniel, and Anna Källén. 2021. I am a Viking! DNA, popular culture and the construction of geneticized identity. *New Genetics and Society* 40: 520–40. [CrossRef]

Tajfel, Henri, and John C. Turner. 1979. An Integrative Theory of Intergroup Conflict. In *The Social Psychology of Intergroup Relations*. Edited by William G. Austin and Stephen Worchel. Monterey: Brooks/Cole, pp. 33–47.

Turner, Marie. 2019. Inclusion and Autism, Belonging. In *Belonging: Rethinking Practices to Support the Well-Being and Identity*. Edited by Annie Guerin and Trish McMenamin. Leiden: Brill Sense, pp. 25–50.

Vaismoradi, Mojtaba, and Sherrill Snelgrove. 2019. Theme in qualitative content analysis and thematic analysis. *FQS, Forum: Qualitative Social Research* 20: 23. [CrossRef]

van Oven, Mannis, and Manfred Kayser. 2008. Updated comprehensive phylogenetic tree of global human mitochondrial DNA variation. *Human Mutation, Mutation in Brief* 30: E386–E394. [CrossRef] [PubMed]

van Oven, Mannis, Anneleen van Geystelen, Manfred Kayser, Ronny Decorte, and Maarten H. D. Larmuseau. 2013. Seeing the wood for the trees: A minimal reference phylogeny for the human Y chromosome. *Human Mutation* 35: 187–91. [CrossRef] [PubMed]

Walker, Jim. 2015. Establishing a sense of belonging for looked after children: The journey from fear and shame to love and belonging. In *Towards Belonging: Negotiating New Relationships for Adopted Children and Those in Care*. Edited by Andrew Briggs. Abingdon: Taylor & Francis, pp. 85–103.

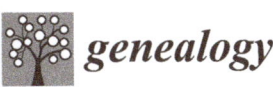

Article

From Human Remains to Powerful Objects: Ancestor Research from a Deep-Time Perspective

Lindsey Büster [1,2]

[1] School of Humanities & Educational Studies, Canterbury Christ Church University, Canterbury CT1 1QU, UK; lindsey.buster@canterbury.ac.uk or lindsey.buster@york.ac.uk
[2] Department of Archaeology, University of York, York YO1 7EP, UK

Abstract: Family history research has seen a surge in popularity in recent years; however, is this preoccupation with who we are and where we come from new? Archaeological evidence suggests that ancestors played crucial and ubiquitous roles in the identities and cosmologies of past societies. This paper will explore how, in the absence of genealogical websites and DNA testing, kinship structures and understandings of personhood beyond genealogy may have influenced concepts of ancestry. Case studies from later prehistoric Britain will demonstrate the ways in which monuments, objects and human remains themselves created bonds between the living and the dead, prompting us to reflect on genealogy as just one aspect of our identity in the present.

Keywords: archaeology; bereavement studies; continuing bonds; problematic stuff; ancestors; personhood

1. Introduction: Ancestors for the Archaeologist

From commercial DNA tests to the rise of genealogy websites and the popularity of TV shows tracing the family trees of celebrities, 'ancestor research' has hit the mainstream in recent years. Archaeologists have long recognized the central role that ancestors played in the lives, and identities, of the living, and the recent increased interest in exploring our 'roots' can perhaps be explained by the highly mobile and globalized societies in which so many of us now live.

Early definitions of ancestors in the anthropological literature perceive them as 'a named, dead forbear [sic] who has living descendants of a designated genealogical class' (Fortes 1965, p. 124), but there are several elements within this definition that require unpicking. Genealogy is defined as 'the history of the past and present members of a family or families' (Cambridge University Press 2022), but need all members of a 'family' necessarily be blood relatives (i.e., determined by DNA)? Indeed, other definitions, such as those based on work among the east African Bantu (Gluckman 1937, p. 125), refer to descendants only as living 'kin', and as this paper will explore, notions of kinship vary widely across the world. Amongst the Lugbara of Uganda (Middleton 1960, p. 33), ancestors can be unnamed, collective and even childless, and 'are not significant *qua* individuals'. Thus, does this focus on the known, named individuals of the (fairly) recent past in our own ancestor research ignore the central role of other types of ancestor (and kin) in the creation and maintenance of social identities? Indeed, the application of the same DNA breakthroughs are revolutionizing our understandings of the prehistoric past, and with it, our understanding of ancestors.

At the broadest scale, ancient genome sequencing has led to the discovery of new early human (hominin) species (Krause et al. 2010; Brown et al. 2016) and unions between these species (Fu et al. 2015; Slon et al. 2018), forcing us to rethink human ancestry at the most fundamental level. Meanwhile, recognition of previously unknown large-scale migrations (Brace et al. 2019; Haak et al. 2015; Olalde et al. 2018, 2019; Patterson et al. 2022)

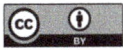

has revealed multiple significant discontinuities in population in various parts of Eurasia over the last several thousand years and requires us to confront the complex relationship between biological and social identity. At the smaller scale, the investigation of Bronze Age intercommunity reproductive exchange (Mittnik et al. 2019) and the reconstruction of Neolithic family trees (Fowler et al. 2022) is giving us insights into the ways in which different kinds of biological and nonbiological relatedness were harnessed within kin groups, while the identification of prehistoric incest (Cassidy et al. 2020) asks us to reconsider culturally-specific taboos and alerts us to the possibility that biological heritage may sometimes be unknown or deliberately hidden.

Even before this scientific revolution, it was clear from the archaeological and ethnographic record that, though ubiquitous, the social roles of ancestors vary widely across time and space. While they may often be known biological relatives with distinct relationships to particular individuals, they may also be envisaged as the more distant progenitors of a whole (perhaps dislocated or fragmented) community. They can also be imagined; particularly in societies in which oral traditions are communicated over many generations and whose cosmologies draw on fuzzier distinctions between humans and the natural world. This paper explores some of the ways in which ancestors have been conceived at different times, in different places, examining in particular how concepts of kin and personhood shape and constrain our understandings of ancestors. I will then explore the ways in which the places, landscapes, objects and the bones of the dead themselves shaped the daily lives of prehistoric communities, and demonstrate that individuals identified by DNA in family history research are but a few of the ancestors we draw on to understand our place in the world around us.

2. Ancestors and Kinship

Closely related to the concept of ancestors are those of kinship and personhood, because the definition and characterisation of the latter two ways of being in the world will influence who, or indeed, what can be considered an ancestor. Because kinship is a socially and culturally constructed expression of 'relationships between people that are based on real or imagined descent' (Darvill 2021, p. 112), it need not correlate directly with biological relatedness. This is indeed one of the challenges of integrating ancient DNA (aDNA) research into archaeological narratives.

At the Neolithic chambered long cairn of Hazleton North in Gloucestershire, UK, dating to c. 3700–3600 cal. BC, recent aDNA analysis of 35 of an estimated 41 individuals has revealed close biological relatedness between 27 people buried in the tomb (Fowler et al. 2022), suggesting a relatively close correlation between biological and social relatedness in this particular community. This is important because many megalithic burial monuments, including Hazleton itself, represent collective tombs in which bodies disarticulate and disintegrate, and through natural processes or manual manipulation by successive generations of descendants, bones eventually become commingled, leading to the interpretation that monuments such as these were designed specifically to facilitate the transformation of known individuals into a communal ancestor. At Hazleton North, however, the bilateral design of the tomb appears to have reflected the kinship structure of its builders; a spatial order that was respected by all five successive generations of interment (with only minor deviations resulting from the collapse of the north passage which blocked the north chamber). This five-generation family was descended from a single male, who had reproduced with four separate women (though we cannot know on present evidence whether the unions were polygamous or represent serial monogamy). Members of the four subsequent sublineages, descended ultimately from the original male and each of the females, were interred together in either the north or south chambers, i.e., two sublineages per chamber. Women who had reproduced with males from this family were present in the tomb, whilst adult lineage daughters were absent, suggesting virilocal burial and female exogamy; a similar finding is suggested by aDNA analysis of a Bronze Age population from the Lech Valley in southern Germany (Mittnik et al. 2019).

Not all sampled individuals were, however, biologically related to the five-generation family at Hazleton North. Biological sons of mothers who also reproduced with lineage males were buried in the tomb, indicating the adoption of half-siblings and step-children into the family, as attested ethnographically by the Nuer of southern Sudan (Stone and King 2019, p. 81). Meanwhile, eight sampled individuals were not biologically-related to any of the other sampled individuals. Three were female and may therefore have been partners of lineage males who either did not reproduce or whose offspring were either not present in the tomb or were not sampled. It is likely, however, that the presence of at least some of these individuals indicates that biological relatedness was not the sole criterion for inclusion in the monument upon death and that other forms of kinship were possible.

The new aDNA analyses at Hazleton North have demonstrated a clear awareness of genealogy, which dictated the design and construction of the burial monument from the outset as well as the maintenance of links with the ancestral dead over at least five generations. Biological relatedness has clearly been a key part of kinship structure for millennia, but there are many other, complementary, ways in which kinship can be perceived and articulated, as we will now explore.

3. Reconsidering 'People'

The centrality of the biologically-bounded individual as the core unit of kinship may in fact be a concept rooted in Western science and philosophy (Robb and Harris 2013; Büster 2018). Personhood refers to the concept of 'what or who was considered to have the capacity of being a person in a given historical context' (Lund 2018) and any universal concept of corporeal identity should not be taken for granted. Indeed, different perceptions of personhood can be found in societies across the globe and may well have existed in the past, particularly in societies where funerary treatments facilitated or even encouraged the commingling of remains (Fowler 2004). In Melanesia, persons are conceived as constituted from a series of parts, which can be separated, exchanged and reconstituted, for example, through the act of gift giving, while in India, persons (particularly ritual practitioners) are considered to be permeable and can be influenced and reconfigured through flows of various substances (Fowler 2004, pp. 7–9; Strathern 1988). Dividual types of personhood such as these are *relational*; that is, they are dependent on the network of relationships between people and, in some cases, things. I suggest that, even within a society in which the bounded individual is the dominant form of personhood, we might see kinship as operating on this same relational level. Indeed, we might even question how universal the concept of the bounded individual is in Western society (Sundberg 2014), when we think, for example, of the capacity for individuals to become 'possessed' by malevolent spirits or overcome by the power of God in certain denominations of Christianity. Even outside of specifically religious contexts, such as our attitudes towards the dead or the processing of grief (Crossland 2010), more dividual aspects of personhood might become elevated, with the capacity for objects (particularly those, such as clothes, which have touched the dead body) to retain some 'essence' of the recently departed or the description of the bereaved as 'filled with grief'. Conversely, the ubiquity of family pets (who often feature in family portraits or as named individuals on Christmas cards) demonstrates that we do not restrict the concept of 'individual' to humans and would have no problem considering these non-biologically-related 'persons' as members of our kin group (Haraway 2003).

In this sense, our perception of kin might conform more to the concept of the 'house society' (Lévi-Strauss 1982), where kin affiliation depends on membership of a particular household rather than biological-relatedness. In some societies, the house *itself* is considered alive and an active ancestor of the household within its walls. Many of the architectural features of the Māori meeting house, for example, were considered to represent parts of the body of an ancestor (veranda = face, porch = brain, ridge-pole = spine, etc.) (van Meijl 1993), with movement along the axis of the house perceived as a progression from past to future (Bradley 2005, p. 51). Among the Batammaliba of Africa (Boivin 2004, p. 7), the clay used to make houses is considered akin to flesh and the plaster applied to the surfaces of walls is referred to as 'skin'. The etymological origins for architectural elements of longhouses ('window' = vidauge = 'wind eye', 'gable' = gavl/geblan = 'head, skull', etc.), together with the 'cremation' and 'burial' of some high-status halls, suggests a similar perception of houses in Viking Scandinavia (Eriksen 2016). Though biological-relatedness is an important part of kinship, it is, for many societies both in the past, and today, only one way in which kinship can be perceived. From flatmates to the family pet, genealogical links are not the only, and not always the strongest, articulation of identity for the living.

4. The House as Ancestor

The Iron Age hillfort of Broxmouth in southeast Scotland was a long-lived settlement, with roughly 800 years of continuous occupation from c. 600 cal. BC to cal. AD 200, over perhaps as many as 32 generations (Armit and McKenzie 2013, p. 513). Roughly one third of the 158 radiocarbon dates obtained for the site indicated redeposited material, out of stratigraphic position (Hamilton et al. 2013), while virtually all of the interior features had been truncated by successive phases of occupation, leaving only the final, Late Iron Age settlement, preserved. This attests to the daily encounters each generation of inhabitants must have had with the material remains of their predecessors, either known, named individuals, or perhaps more communal ancestors. Indeed, one of the Late Iron Age (Phase 6) roundhouses seems to have been sited and oriented in relation to a Phase 1 burial interred some 20 generations earlier (Büster and Armit 2021, p. 30, Figure 4.2).

The Late Iron Age phase of the settlement, dating from c. 100 cal. BC to cal. AD 155, consisted of eight surviving roundhouses of timber and stone, including several structures (Houses 4, 5 and 7) which had undergone systematic remodeling on a number of occasions. House 4, the best preserved, had seen five stages of modification on a roughly generational or bigenerational basis (i.e., every 25 to 40 years) (Büster 2021a, p. 667, Figure 5). The modifications were not structurally necessary, and each time, rather than reusing the previous fabric, the new structure was built *inside* the shell of its predecessor, resulting in successive arcs of concentric walling and paved floors laid one on top of the other, ultimately reducing the final footprint to less than 40% of its original size. Furthermore, during each rebuild, objects were placed between the wall faces, under the paved floors and inside pits before their infilling, quickly becoming hidden from view as construction progressed. The types of objects chosen, and their placement within the building, appeared to reference one another across the generations: a bone 'spoon' placed under the stage 1 wall was mirrored by a second, tucked under the stage 5 wall, five or more generations later; quernstones for grinding grain (deposited upside down with their grinding faces deliberately smashed away) were repeatedly placed towards the rear of the structure, and very often over the infilled pits. It has been suggested (Campbell 1991, p. 133) that the feeder pipes of rotary quernstones would have facilitated, for example, the pouring of votive libations into the features below (Büster 2021a, p. 669, Figure 8), creating tangible links with previous structures and any ancestral spirits thought to reside within them. Certainly, a similar phenomenon existed at the first-century BC cemetery complex of Goeblingen-Nospelt in Luxembourg, where a large ceramic vessel (known as a dolium) was placed over the grave chamber of a high-status female and, having had its base removed, formed the focus for votive offerings for at least 175 years (Metzler and Gaeng 2009; Fernández-Götz 2016, p. 175, Figure 9). In an increasingly mobile and global world, it is unlikely that many inhabitants of a particular house will represent the fifth generation of their family to have lived there. What Broxmouth shows us, however, is the power of past generations (known, unknown, real or imagined) to shape the world in which we find ourselves and that feelings of responsibility towards their remembrance are ubiquitous and deeply rooted.

5. Redefining Ancestors

The deposition of human bone (the physical remains of ancestors) within roundhouses is not uncommon. In House 4 at Broxmouth, described above, cranial and mandible fragments from separate individuals were deposited at the base of the stage 2 wall before it was sealed during construction of the stage 4 roundhouse. The condition of these human remains relative to the faunal bone which accompanied them suggests that they had been curated prior to deposition (Büster and Armit 2021, p. 33). A similar phenomenon can be found at Cnip, Lewis, Scotland, where, sometime in the first century AD, a human cranium, together with a pot sherd and a stone mimicking the shape of the cranium, were placed into a scoop dug prior to paving of the floor of a small building appended to an earlier structure (Armit 2006, p. 58). The human bone appeared to be weathered, suggesting that it had spent time elsewhere before deposition, but in this instance, subsequent radiocarbon dating (to 1540–1410 cal. BC; Armit and Shapland 2015, p. 42) indicated that it predated the structure by more than a millennium and a half and was likely derived from a Middle Bronze Age cemetery a few hundred metres away (Dunwell et al. 1995). We cannot know whether the cranium was deliberately exhumed from the cemetery or whether it was a chance find, having eroded out of the sand over the intervening 60 generations, but it is likely that, as with the Phase 1 burial outside Late Iron Age House 2 at Broxmouth, this 'ancestor' (if this is indeed how they were perceived) had passed into the realm of mythical time (Gosden and Lock 1998).

A more overt example of interaction with the long dead may be represented by two individuals buried under the floor of a Late Bronze Age roundhouse at Cladh Hallan, South Uist, Outer Hebrides, Scotland. A combination of osteological, isotopic, aDNA and histological evidence (Parker Pearson et al. 2005, 2007; Hanna et al. 2012; Booth et al. 2015) revealed that both individuals were composites of three people (i.e., six in total) and were subject to mummification processes which may have utilised the acidic and anaerobic conditions of nearby peat bogs. Both bodies appear to have spent considerable time in other contexts, perhaps above ground amongst the living, as the radiocarbon dates of their various skeletal elements considerably predate their Late Bronze Age depositional context. Indeed, there is no overlap between the cranial and postcranial elements of one of the 'mummies', who appears to be a composite of individuals who would never have known in each other in life, and who died several hundred years before construction of the roundhouses which served as their final resting place.

Interaction with 'mummy bundles' of the long dead is also evidenced at the Sculptor's Cave in northeast Scotland (Armit and Büster 2020); a rare example of a surviving funerary population from Late Bronze Age and Iron Age Britain in a period when the dead become virtually invisible archaeologically (Harding 2016, p. 4). This remote sea cave, on the south coast of the Moray Firth, formed the focus for funerary and ritual activity over roughly 1500 years, in a landscape that had itself been a place of the dead since the Neolithic (c. 4000 BC) (Büster et al. 2020). At an adjacent cave, Early Bronze Age (c. 2400–2200 BC) human remains were redeposited in sediments associated with Late Bronze Age (c. 1100–800 BC) funerary activity, indicating close engagement with and manipulation of ancestors (Büster and Armit 2016). At the Sculptor's Cave, evidence for Iron Age visitors is attested by thick accumulated deposits including structures, grain processing waste and hearths for the preparation and cooking of meals. This suggests frequent visits to and provision for the ancestral dead, who (thanks to earlier funerary treatment and the exceptional preservational qualities of the salty cave environment) may have resembled something akin to mummy bundles (Armit and Büster 2020, p. 251), dressed in finery such as the gold-covered hair rings later gathered together and deposited as a cache at the furthest recess of the cave.

Caves themselves are known, from prehistory to present, to be liminal places between worlds and would therefore have been appropriate places for communion with the ancestral otherworld (Büster et al. 2019). After a further 1500 years of visitation, including more funerary activity in the Roman Iron Age (c. first to fourth centuries AD), the ancestral power of the cave was harnessed in another dramatic way, as the arena for the execution of up to nine individuals by decapitation sometime in the third century AD (Armit and Büster 2020, pp. 253–55). While it would have been much more practical to execute these, presumably unwilling, victims at the nearest settlement, or even on the cliff top, surrounded by a large audience, it was felt necessary to escort them on the arduous journey down the cliff and across the rocky foreshore to the cave itself. The Sculptor's Cave, and its ancestral inhabitants, must therefore have been crucial to the event—either for legitimising this violent act or as witness to the desecration of a long-sacred landscape.

Whatever the precise circumstances, funerary activity at the cave ceased shortly afterwards, sometime in the fourth century AD (Hamilton et al. 2020). One of the last visible acts was the carving of a series of symbols around the cave's distinct twin entrance passages in the Pictish period (c. sixth to eighth centuries AD, but perhaps as early as the fifth century based on emerging evidence elsewhere in Scotland; Noble et al. 2018). This pictographic writing system, which rarely occurs in caves and is more commonly found on freestanding 'symbol stones', has not yet been 'decoded', but one interpretation is that the symbols, which often occur in pairs (as at the Sculptor's Cave), represent two-part personal names (Samson 1992; Forsyth 1995). It is possible that the symbols merely represent attempts by a newly Christianised community to warn people away from or symbolically close off a dangerous pagan place ('strewn with human bones', as the original excavator found it in 1927; Benton 1931, p. 177), or, if they really were names and carved within a century of the decapitation event, they may represent a memorial to the fallen who died within living memory. Though we cannot know the precise meaning of the carvings, it is clear that this ancestral place, which necessitated constant visitation over more than a millennium, had now become somewhere to avoid, and this reminds us that encounters with ancestors are not always welcomed and that they can bring about negative and unwanted feelings.

6. Reimagining Ancestors

Caves are often the sites of enduring funerary and ritual activity. We have already considered their liminal nature, but the fact that they are hewn from solid rock makes them durable places in the landscape. In fact, in some societies, stone is considered representative of the dead (and the ancestors) themselves. In Madagascar, for example, biological and social ageing is conceptualised as a kind of 'hardening' (Bloch 1995a, 1995b, p. 215), and so wood is reserved for the construction of houses for the living, while stone is used for tombs and for standing stones perceived as portals for communication with the dead (Parker Pearson and Ramilisonina 1998, p. 311). Among the San peoples of South Africa and Indigenous communities in Australia, the dulling and darkening of rock carvings through weathering is thought to indicate the reclaiming of images by the spirit world, and frequent recarving and repainting is required to maintain these communication channels with ancestors (Ouzman 2001; Taçon 2004, p. 39). If we view the Late Iron Age roundhouses at Broxmouth through this lens, perhaps the periodic remodeling of the structures, in which timber elements were gradually replaced in stone (as in House 5) or the encasing of one house within the stone shell of its predecessor (as in Houses 4 and 7), was similarly seen as a kind of biological 'hardening' and was a tangible cue to the longevity of the household within. Likewise, remodeling of the structures, and the deposition of particular objects, may have been considered necessary to maintain links with genealogical ancestors.

Certainly, the caching of objects within the walls of House 4 at Broxmouth would have been central to the biography of each household; the stories passed down about now-hidden objects and their owners constituting an important part of their identity. Objects are powerful mnemonic devices. We see this, literally 'at play', in House 4, with the curation of two distinctive gaming pieces deposited at the base of the stage 2 wall with the human bone fragments during construction of stage 4 roundhouse; their partner was deposited in a large pit during remodeling of the stage 2 roundhouse several generations earlier (Büster and Armit 2013, pp. 138–52). These personal and highly tactile items, perhaps still played with, would have represented a tangible link to past events and deceased relatives in much the same way that heirlooms do today. The recollection of specific details about the nature and location of long-buried artefacts over multiple generations may seem like a stretch in communities who could not rely on photographs or written documents, but ethnographic evidence attests to the transmission of genealogical histories, and even the names of houses

(Best 1927, p. 96), over periods of between 500 and 700 years (Ballard 1994); more than sufficient to encompass the time which lapsed between, for example, the deposition of the paired bone spoons under the walls of the first and last iterations of House 4. Family history research is a popular hobby and pastime today but tends to be undertaken by lone individuals sifting silently through archival documents or ancestry websites. In the past, and in many societies around the world today, however, the transmission of genealogical narratives would have been a core part of everyday life, with song, dance and stories told and retold in communal settings, and perhaps even in the presence of ancestors themselves.

7. Ancestors and Objects

There is of course a paradox in the interpretation of the cached objects in House 4 at Broxmouth. If objects were so fundamental to the maintenance of 'continuing bonds'[1] with the dead, then why do we find them cached so often in the archaeological record? Whether a grave or a midden, it is, after all, the stuff that people throw away, those things taken out of circulation amongst the world of the living, that are left behind for us to find. Furthermore, why do we so often find these items deposited in such unusual ways in the houses of Iron Age Britain? Indeed, this phenomenon is so common on later prehistoric settlements in Britain that it has its own classificatory category: 'structured deposit'. Originally coined in specific reference to the spatial patterning of pottery, flint and bone at Neolithic causewayed enclosures (Richards and Thomas 1984), structured deposition is now commonly used to describe any deposit which appears to represent the deliberate deposition of material in nonfunerary contexts (Garrow 2012). The use of different classificatory terms for cached objects in funerary and nonfunerary contexts is an important one, reflecting the different trajectories of each subdiscipline within archaeology. It has, however, as I have suggested elsewhere (Büster 2021b), hindered interpretation of this latter category of material.

During research on the ways in which archaeology can encourage discussions around the often-taboo topic of death, dying and bereavement in the UK today (Croucher et al. 2020), many of the group discussions I helped facilitate focused not on the dead body itself but the objects left behind. On several occasions, it became clear that these objects were not, as we might think of grave goods in the archaeological record, treasured heirlooms with long biographies serving as mnemonic devices for cherished moments. An old pair of worn out and misshapen shoes provoked memories of an individual past their prime, while a jar of Horlicks (a powdered malted drink) had been acquired during a routine shopping trip and gifted to the bereaved only days before their relative's death (Büster 2021b, pp. 976, 981). Overnight, the jar of Horlicks 'became like an artefact' and hugely problematic for the bereaved individual; they did not like Horlicks and perhaps they would not have felt comfortable drinking it in any case, but despite this, they could not bring themselves to throw it out with the routine rubbish of daily life, and it stayed in the cupboard for five years until it became solid. The owner of both the shoes and the Horlicks did eventually throw these items away, citing respectively that 'it was a sign of getting through the grief' and that 'you have to hold onto things until it's time to release them' (Büster 2021b, pp. 976, 981).

The rise of 'death cleaning' movements (Magnusson 2017), where people are encouraged to sort out their affairs long before their death, and the increasing popularity of 'tidying experts' (e.g., Kondo 2014), suggest that these are not isolated stories and that 'problematic stuff' (Büster 2021b) need not be restricted to the belongings of the dead. Indeed, there are attics, cupboards, garages and basements bursting with cassette tapes from teenage years that can no longer be played and baby clothes that no longer fit. This material represents the problematic stuff not of the physical dead, but the socially dead personae of the living. Humans are very good at making things—it is perhaps what makes us human in the first place—but the constant creation and/or acquisition of stuff is emotionally heavy, and throwing away *some* things is difficult; it requires special processing outside of the normal practice of waste disposal.

This poses a particular problem for the later prehistoric communities of Britain. Funerals are highly structured and ritualised events, which means that graves make good places to deposit problematic stuff. As noted previously, however, the majority of the later prehistoric dead in Britain are invisible archaeologically. The general absence of human remains and their weathered and isolated nature when found (usually as part of structured deposits) suggests that excarnation by exposure (during which the body is left to naturally disarticulate and disperse; Carr and Knüsel 1997) was probably the majority rite. If this was the case, there was no *body* to bury, no need for a grave pit, and thus no appropriate context in which to deposit problematic stuff. It may, therefore, be the case that structured deposits (that is, cached objects in pits and in other formalised contexts such as roundhouses) are the grave goods of later prehistoric Britain, but that prioritisation of the physical human body in our interpretations has led us to overlook them as such. As outlined earlier, foregrounding the bounded individual in this way may, in fact, be a relatively recent and culturally-specific perception of the world. In fact, objects have the potential to be as, if not more, emotionally powerful than the physical dead, *particularly* in those societies where the living are detached from post-mortem care and funerary treatment of the dead body. Acknowledging this fact does not make objects any less problematic for us in the present, but it helps us understand that the visceral reactions evoked by certain objects at certain times are an inevitable and enduring part of grief.

8. Conclusions: Living with Ancestors

It has been suggested that 'there are too many ancestors in contemporary archaeological interpretation, and they are being asked to do too much' (Whitley 2002, p. 119). The study of ancestors, however, lies at the heart of archaeology, history and allied disciplines, and in this sense, everything we study is 'ancestral'. As we have seen, from attempts to arrest the decomposition process in the Bronze Age 'mummies' at Cladh Hallan to current ethical debates over the digital legacies of the deceased (with the estimated 30 million legacy profiles on Facebook exceeding the number of living users), ancestors, in various forms, have always formed a central part of our understandings of the world and continue to play fundamental roles in the lives of the living. Though they can be used for positive effect, their continued presence is not always welcomed (as attested by the challenge of disposing of 'problematic stuff'), and the current rise of populist, nationalist agendas is once again seeing their misappropriation and misuse for contemporary political ends (Bonacchi forthcoming). The deep-time and global perspective presented here demonstrates that our relationships with ancestors are complex and multi-faceted, that concepts of ancestor and kin are culturally and contextually specific, and, that whether positive or negative, comforting or problematic, ancestors are an ever-present and ubiquitous part of life.

Funding: This research received no external funding.

Institutional Review Board Statement: Not applicable.

Informed Consent Statement: Not applicable.

Data Availability Statement: Not applicable.

Conflicts of Interest: The author declares no conflict of interest.

Notes

[1] Continuing bonds is a theory developed in contemporary studies of death, dying and bereavement (Klass et al. 1996; Stroebe et al. 2012; Walter 1996). It grew from dissatisfaction with traditional models of grief which emphasised the need for detachment from the deceased (Freud 1917), or asserted that the grieving process progressed through a unilinear series of stages towards the restoration of a pre-bereavement status quo (Kubler-Ross 1969; Bowlby 1973, 1980; Worden 1991). Grief, in practice, is far more complex than a linear trajectory of 'recovery', and (consciously or unconsciously) individuals often form new types of relationships ('continuing bonds') that endure to a greater or lesser extent throughout the rest of their lives (Shuchter and Zisook 1993, p. 34).

References

Armit, Ian. 2006. *Anatomy of an Iron Age Roundhouse: The Cnip Wheelhouse Excavations, Lewis*. Edinburgh: Society of Antiquaries of Scotland, p. 58, Illustration 2.26, ISBN 978-090-390-332-5.

Armit, Ian, and Lindsey Büster. 2020. *Darkness Visible. The Sculptor's Cave, NE Scotland: From the Bronze Age to the Picts*. Edinburgh: Society of Antiquaries of Scotland, ISBN 978-190-833-217-2.

Armit, Ian, and Jo McKenzie. 2013. *An Inherited Place: Broxmouth Hillfort and the South-East Scottish Iron Age*. Edinburgh: Society of Antiquaries of Scotland, ISBN 978-190-833-205-9.

Armit, Ian, and Fiona Shapland. 2015. Death and display in the North Atlantic: The Bronze and Iron Age Human Remains from Cnip, Lewis, Outer Hebrides. *Journal of the North Atlantic* 9: 35–44. [CrossRef]

Ballard, Chris. 1994. The centre cannot hold: Trade networks and sacred geography in the Papua New Guinea highlands. *Archaeology in Oceania* 29: 130–48. [CrossRef]

Benton, Sylvia. 1931. The excavation of the Sculptor's Cave, Covesea, Morayshire. *Proceedings of the Society of Antiquaries of Scotland* 65: 177–216. [CrossRef]

Best, Eldon. 1927. *The Pa Māori*. Dominion Museum Bulletin 6. Wellington: Whitcombe and Tombs Ltd., p. 96, ISBN 978-187-738-508-7.

Bloch, Maurice. 1995a. The resurrection of the house amongst the Zafimaniry of Madagascar. In *About the House: Lévi-Strauss and Beyond*. Edited by Janet Carsten and Stephen Hugh-Jones. Cambridge: Cambridge University Press, pp. 69–83, ISBN 978-052-147-953-0.

Bloch, Maurice. 1995b. Questions not to be asked of Malagasy carvings. In *Interpreting Archaeology: Finding Meaning in the Past*. Edited by Ian Hodder, Michael Shanks, Victor Buchli, John Carman, Jonathan Last and Gavin Lucas. London: Routledge, pp. 212–15, ISBN 978-041-515-744-5.

Boivin, Nicole. 2004. From veneration to exploitation: Human engagement with the mineral world. In *Soils, Stones and Symbols: Cultural Perceptions of the Mineral World*. Edited by Nicole Boivin and Mary Ann Owoc. London: UCL Press, pp. 1–29, ISBN 978-184-472-039-2.

Bonacchi, Chiara. Forthcoming. *Heritage and Nationalism: Understanding Populism through Big Data*. London: UCL Press, ISBN 978-178-735-803-4.

Booth, Thomas J., Andrew T. Chamberlain, and Mike Parker Pearson. 2015. Mummification in Bronze Age Britain. *Antiquity* 89: 1155–73. [CrossRef]

Bowlby, John. 1973. *Attachment and Loss: Separation, Anxiety and Anger*. London: Hogarth, vol. II, ISBN 978-071-266-621-3.

Bowlby, John. 1980. *Attachment and Loss: Sadness and Depression*. London: Hogarth, vol. III, ISBN 978-070-120-350-4.

Brace, Selina, Yoan Diekmann, Thomas J. Booth, Lucy van Dorp, Zuzana Faltyskova, Nadin Rohland, Swapan Mallick, Iñigo Olalde, Matthew Ferry, Megan Michel, and et al. 2019. Ancient genomes indicate population replacement in Early Neolithic Britain. *Nature Ecology & Evolution* 3: 765–71.

Bradley, Richard. 2005. *Ritual and Domestic in Prehistoric Europe*. London: Routledge, p. 51, ISBN 978-041-534-551-4.

Brown, Samantha, Thomas Higham, Viviane Slon, Svante Pääbo, Matthias Meyer, Katerina Douka, Fiona Brock, Daniel Comeskey, Noemi Procopio, Michael Shunkov, and et al. 2016. Identification of a new hominin bone from Denisova Cave, Siberia using collagen fingerprinting and mitochondrial DNA analysis. *Nature Scientific Reports* 6: 23559. [CrossRef]

Büster, Lindsey. 2018. Bodies and embodiment. In *The SAS Encyclopedia of Archaeological Sciences*. Edited by Sandra L. Lopez Varela. Hoboken: John Wiley & Sons, vol. II, pp. 1–5, ISBN 978-0-470-67461-1. [CrossRef]

Büster, Lindsey. 2021a. Iron Age mnemonics: A biographical approach to dwelling in later prehistoric Britain. *Cambridge Archaeological Journal* 31: 661–74. [CrossRef]

Büster, Lindsey. 2021b. Problematic stuff: Death, memory and the reinterpretation of cached objects. *Antiquity* 95: 973–85. [CrossRef]

Büster, Lindsey, and Ian Armit. 2013. Phase 6: The Late Iron Age village. In *An Inherited Place: Broxmouth Hillfort and the South-East Scottish Iron Age*. Edinburgh: Society of Antiquaries of Scotland, pp. 115–86, ISBN 978-190-833-205-9.

Büster, Lindsey, and Ian Armit. 2016. *The Covesea Caves Project: Fieldwork 2015 Data Structure Report (December 2016)*. Unpublished Report. Bradford: University of Bradford.

Büster, Lindsey, and Ian Armit. 2021. Materialising memories: Inheritance, performance and practice at Broxmouth hillfort, south-east Scotland. In *Gardening Time: Reflections on Memory, Monuments and History in Scotland and Sardinia*. Edited by Simon Stoddart, Ethan D. Aines and Caroline Malone. Cambridge: McDonald Institute for Archaeological Research, pp. 27–36, ISBN 978-1-913344-04-7.

Büster, Lindsey, Eugène Warmenbol, and Dimitrij Mlekuž. 2019. Between worlds: Bridging the divide between method and theory in understanding the ritual use of caves in later prehistory. In *Between Worlds: Understanding Ritual Cave Use in Later Prehistory*. Edited by Lindsey Büster, Eugène Warmenbol and Dimitrij Mlekuž. New York: Springer, pp. 1–6, ISBN 978-331-999-021-7, ISBN 978-331-999-022-4.

Büster, Lindsey, Ian Armit, and Alex Fitzpatrick. 2020. New light on the Covesea Caves, north-east Scotland. *PAST* 96: 2–5.

Cambridge University Press. 2022. Cambridge Advanced Learner's Dictionary & Thesaurus. Available online: https://dictionary.cambridge.org/dictionary/english/genealogy (accessed on 21 February 2022).

Campbell, Ewan. 1991. Excavations of a wheelhouse and other Iron Age structures at Sollas, North Uist, by R.J.C. Atkinson in 1957. *Proceedings of the Society of Antiquaries of Scotland* 121: 117–73.

Carr, Gillian, and Christopher Knüsel. 1997. The ritual framework of excarnation by exposure as the mortuary practice of the Early and Middle Iron Ages of central southern Britain. In *Reconstructing Iron Age Societies*. Edited by Adam Gwilt and Colin Haselgrove. Oxford: Oxbow Books, pp. 167–73, ISBN 978-190-018-804-3.

Cassidy, Lara M., Ros Ó Maoldúin, Thomas Kador, Ann Lynch, Carleton Jones, Peter C. Woodman, Eileen Murphy, Greer Ramsey, Marion Dowd, Alice Noonan, and et al. 2020. A dynastic elite in monumental Neolithic society. *Nature* 582: 384–88. [CrossRef] [PubMed]

Crossland, Zoë. 2010. Materiality and embodiment. In *The Oxford Handbook of Material Culture Studies*. Edited by Dan Hicks and Mary C. Beaudry. Oxford: Oxford University Press, pp. 386–405, ISBN 978-019-921-871-4.

Croucher, Karina, Lindsey Büster, Jennifer Dayes, Laura Green, Justine Raynsford, Louise Comerford Boyes, and Christina Faull. 2020. Archaeology and contemporary death: Using the past to provoke, challenge and engage. *PLoS ONE* 15: e0244058. [CrossRef] [PubMed]

Darvill, Timothy. 2021. *The Concise Oxford Dictionary of Archaeology*, 3rd ed. Oxford: Oxford University Press, p. 112, ISBN 978-019-172-713-9.

Dunwell, Andrew, Tim Neighbour, and Trevor G. Cowie. 1995. A cist burial adjacent to the Bronze Age burial at Cnip, Uig, Isle of Lewis. *Proceedings of the Society of Antiquaries of Scotland* 125: 279–88.

Eriksen, Marianne Hem. 2016. Commemorating dwelling: The death and burial of houses in Iron and Viking Age Scandinavia. *European Journal of Archaeology* 19: 477–96. [CrossRef]

Fernández-Götz, Manuel. 2016. The power of the past: Ancestral cult and collective memory in the central European Iron Age. In *Funerary Practices during the Bronze and Iron Ages in Central and Southeast Europe, Proceedings of the 14th International Colloquium of Funerary Archaeology in Čačak, Serbia, 24th–27th September 2015*. Edited by Valeriu Sîrbu, Miloš Jevtić, Katarina Dmitrović and Marija Ljuština. Čačak: Boegard, pp. 165–78, ISBN 978-866-427-040-3.

Forsyth, Katherine. 1995. Some thoughts on Pictish symbols as a formal writing system. In *The Worm, the Germ and the Thorn: Pictish and Related Studies Presented to Isabel Henderson*. Edited by Isabel Henderson and David Henry. Brechin: Pinkfoot Press, pp. 85–98, ISBN 978-187-401-216-0.

Fortes, Meyer. 1965. Some reflections on ancestor worship in Africa. In *African Systems of Thought*. Edited by Meyer Fortes and Germaine Dieterlen. London: Oxford University Press for The International African Institute, pp. 122–42, ISBN 978-081-306-251-8.

Fowler, Chris. 2004. *The Archaeology of Personhood: An Anthropological Approach*. London: Routledge, ISBN 978-041-531-722-1.

Fowler, Chris, Iñigo Olalde, Vicki Cummings, Ian Armit, Lindsey Büster, Sarah Cuthbert, Nadin Rohland, Olivia Cheronet, Ron Pinhasi, and David Reich. 2022. Complex kinship practices revealed in a five-generation family from Neolithic Britain. *Nature* 601: 584–87. [CrossRef]

Freud, Sigmund. 1917. Mourning and melancholia. In *The Standard Complete Psychological Works of Sigmund Freud*. Edited by James Strachey. London: Hogarth, vol. 14, pp. 237–58, ISBN 978-070-120-067-1.

Fu, Qiaomei, Mateja Hajdinjak, Oana Teodora Moldovan, Silviu Constantin, Swapan Mallick, Pontus Skoglund, Nick Patterson, Nadin Rohland, Iosif Lazaridis, Birgit Nickel, and et al. 2015. An early modern human from Romania with a recent Neanderthal ancestor. *Nature* 524: 216–19. [CrossRef]

Garrow, Duncan. 2012. Odd deposits and average practice: A critical history of the concept of structured deposition. *Archaeological Dialogues* 19: 85–115. [CrossRef]

Gluckman, Max. 1937. Mortuary customs and the belief in survival after death among the south-eastern Bantu. *Bantu Studies* 11: 117–36. [CrossRef]

Gosden, Chris, and Gary Lock. 1998. Prehistoric histories. *World Archaeology* 30: 2–12. [CrossRef]

Haak, Wolfgang, Iosif Lazaridis, Nick Patterson, Nadin Rohland, Swapan Mallick, Bastien Llamas, Guido Brandt, Susanne Nordenfelt, Eadaoin Harney, Kristin Stewardson, and et al. 2015. Massive migration from the steppe was a source for Indo-European languages in Europe. *Nature* 522: 207–11. [CrossRef]

Hamilton, Derek, Jo McKenzie, Ian Armit, and Lindsey Büster. 2013. Chronology: Radiocarbon dating and Bayesian modelling. In *An Inherited Place: Broxmouth Hillfort and the South-East Scottish Iron Age*. Edinburgh: Society of Antiquaries of Scotland, pp. 191–224, ISBN 978-190-833-205-9.

Hamilton, Derek, Ian Armit, Rick Schulting, and Lindsey Büster. 2020. Chronology: Archaeology, radiocarbon dating and Bayesian modelling. In *Darkness Visible. The Sculptor's Cave, NE Scotland: From the Bronze Age to the Picts*. Edinburgh: Society of Antiquaries of Scotland, pp. 75–86, ISBN 978-190-833-217-2.

Hanna, Jayd, Abigail S. Bouwman, Keri A. Brown, Mike Parker Pearson, and Terrence A. Brown. 2012. Ancient DNA typing shows that a Bronze Age mummy is a composite of different skeletons. *Journal of Archaeological Science* 39: 2774–79. [CrossRef]

Haraway, Donna. 2003. *The Companion Species Manifesto: Dogs, People, and Significant Otherness*. Chicago: Prickly Paradigm Press, ISBN 978-097-175-758-5.

Harding, Dennis W. 2016. *Death and Burial in Iron Age Britain*. Oxford: Oxford University Press, p. 4, ISBN 978-019-968-756-5.

Klass, Dennis, Phyllis R. Silverman, and Steven L. Nickman, eds. 1996. *Continuing Bonds: New Understandings of Grief*. London: Taylor and Francis, ISBN 978-156-032-339-6.

Kondo, Marie. 2014. *The Life-Changing Magic of Tidying Up: The Japanese Art of Decluttering and Organizing*. Berkeley: Ten Speed Press, ISBN 978-160-774-730-7.

Krause, Johannes, Qiaomei Fu, Jeffrey M. Good, Bence Viola, Michael V. Shunkov, Anatoli P. Derevianko, and Svante Pääbo. 2010. The complete mitochondrial DNA genome of an unknown hominin from southern Siberia. *Nature* 464: 894–97. [CrossRef] [PubMed]

Kubler-Ross, Elisabeth. 1969. *On Death and Dying*. New York: Macmillan, ISBN 978-002-605-060-9.

Lévi-Strauss, Claude. 1982. *The Way of the Masks*. Translated by Sylvia Modelski. Seattle: University of Washington Press, ISBN 978-029-596-636-6.

Lund, Julie. 2018. Personhood and objecthood. In *The SAS Encyclopedia of Archaeological Sciences*. Edited by Sandra L. Lopez Varela. Hoboken: John Wiley & Sons, vol. II, pp. 1–4, ISBN 978-0-470-67461-1. [CrossRef]

Magnusson, Margareta. 2017. *The Gentle Art of Swedish Death Cleaning: How to Free Yourself and Your Family from a Lifetime of Clutter*. Edinburgh: Canongate Books, ISBN 978-178-689-108-2.

Metzler, Jeannot, and Catherine Gaeng. 2009. *Goeblange-Nospelt: Une Nécropole Aristocratique Trévire*. Luxembourg: Musée National d'Histoire et d'Art, Dossiers d'Archéologie du Musée National d'Histoire et d'Art, vol. 13, pp. 501–8, ISBN 978-287-985-065-8.

Middleton, John. 1960. *Lugbara Religion: Ritual and Authority among an East African People*. London: Oxford University Press for The International African Institute, ISBN 978-019-724-136-3.

Mittnik, Alissa, Ken Massy, Corina Knipper, Fabian Wittenborn, Ronny Friedrich, Saskia Pfrengle, Marta Burri, Nadine Carlichi-Witjes, Heidi Deeg, Anja Furtwängler, and et al. 2019. Kinship-based social inequality in Bronze Age Europe. *Science* 366: 731–34. [CrossRef] [PubMed]

Noble, Gordon, Martin Goldberg, and Derek Hamilton. 2018. The development of the Pictish symbol system: Inscribing identity beyond the edges of Empire. *Antiquity* 92: 1329–48. [CrossRef]

Olalde, Iñigo, Selina Brace, Morton E. Allentoft, Ian Armit, Kristian Kristiansen, Thomas Booth, Nadin Rohland, Swapan Mallick, Anna Szécsényi-Nagy, Alissa Mittnik, and et al. 2018. The Beaker phenomenon and the genomic transformation of northwest Europe. *Nature* 255: 190–96. [CrossRef] [PubMed]

Olalde, Iñigo, Swapan Mallick, Nick Patterson, Nadin Rohland, Vanessa Villalba-Mouco, Marina Silva, Katharina Dulias, Ceiridwen J. Edwards, Francesca Gandini, Maria Pala, and et al. 2019. The genomic history of the Iberian Peninsula over the past 8000 years. *Science* 363: 1230–1234. [CrossRef]

Ouzman, Sven. 2001. Seeing is deceiving: Rock art and the non-visual. *World Archaeology* 33: 237–56. [CrossRef]

Parker Pearson, Mike, and Ramilisonina. 1998. Stonehenge for the ancestors: The stones pass on the message. *Antiquity* 72: 308–26. [CrossRef]

Parker Pearson, Mike, Andrew Chamberlain, Oliver Craig, Peter Marshall, Jacqui Mulville, Helen Smith, Carolyn Chenery, Matthew Collins, Gordon Cook, Geoffrey Craig, and et al. 2005. Evidence for mummification in Bronze Age Britain. *Antiquity* 79: 529–46. [CrossRef]

Parker Pearson, Mike, Andrew Chamberlain, Matthew Collins, Christie Cox, Geoffrey Craig, Oliver Craig, Jen Hiller, Peter Marshall, Jacqui Mulville, and Helen Smith. 2007. Further evidence for mummification in Bronze Age Britain. *Antiquity* 81. Available online: http://www.antiquity.ac.uk/projgall/parker312/ (accessed on 6 January 2022).

Patterson, Nick, Michael Isakov, Thomas Booth, Lindsey Büster, Claire-Elise Fischer, Iñigo Olalde, Harald Ringbauer, Ali Akbari, Olivia Cheronet, Madeleine Bleasdale, and et al. 2022. Large-scale migration into Britain during the Middle to Late Bronze Age. *Nature* 601: 588–94. [CrossRef] [PubMed]

Richards, Colin, and Julian Thomas. 1984. Ritual activity and structured deposition in later Neolithic Wessex. In *Neolithic Studies: A Review of Some Current Research*. Edited by Richard Bradley and Julie Gardiner. Oxford: British Archaeological Reports (British Series), vol. 133, pp. 189–218, ISBN 978-086-054-291-9.

Robb, John, and Oliver J. T. Harris. 2013. *The Body in History: Europe from the Palaeolithic to the Future*. Cambridge: Cambridge University Press, ISBN 978-052-119-528-7.

Samson, Ross. 1992. The reinterpretation of the Pictish symbols. *Journal of the British Archaeological Association* 145: 29–65. [CrossRef]

Shuchter, Stephen R., and Sidney Zisook. 1993. The course of normal grief. In *Handbook of Bereavement: Theory, Research, and Intervention*. Edited by Margaret S. Stroebe, Wolfgang Stroebe and Robert O. Hansson. Cambridge: Cambridge University Press, pp. 23–43, ISBN 978-052-144-853-6.

Slon, Viviane, Fabrizio Mafessoni, Benjamin Vernot, Cesare de Filippo, Steffi Grote, Bence Viola, Mateja Hajdinjak, Stéphane Peyrégne, Sarah Nagel, Samantha Brown, and et al. 2018. The genome of the offspring of a Neanderthal mother and a Denisovan father. *Nature* 561: 113–16. [CrossRef]

Stone, Linda, and Diane E. King. 2019. *Kinship and Gender: An Introduction*, 6th ed. New York: Routledge, p. 81, ISBN 978-081-335-094-3.

Strathern, Marilyn. 1988. *The Gender of the Gift: Problems with Women and Problems with Society in Melanesia*. Berkeley: University of California Press, ISBN 978-052-007-202-2.

Stroebe, Margaret S., Georgios Abakoumkin, Wolfgang Stroebe, and Henk Schut. 2012. Continuing bonds in adjustment to bereavement: Impact of abrupt versus gradual separation. *Personal Relationships* 19: 255–66. [CrossRef]

Sundberg, Juanita. 2014. Decolonizing posthumanist geographies. *Cultural Geographies* 21: 33–47. [CrossRef]

Taçon, Paul S. C. 2004. Ochre, clay, stone and art: The symbolic importance of minerals as life-force among Aboriginal peoples of northern and central Australia. In *Soils, Stones and Symbols: Cultural Perceptions of the Mineral World*. Edited by Nicole Boivin and Mary Ann Owoc. London: UCL Press, pp. 31–42, ISBN 978-184-472-039-2.

van Meijl, Toon. 1993. Māori meeting-houses in and over time. In *Inside Austronesian Houses: Perspectives on Domestic Designs for Living*. Edited by James J. Fox. Canberra: Australian National University, pp. 194–218, ISBN 978-073-151-595-0.

Walter, Tony. 1996. A new model of grief: Bereavement and biography. *Mortality* 1: 7–25. [CrossRef]
Whitley, James. 2002. Too many ancestors. *Antiquity* 76: 119–26. [CrossRef]
Worden, J. William. 1991. *Grief Counseling and Grief Therapy: A Handbook for the Mental Health Practitioner*. New York: Springer.

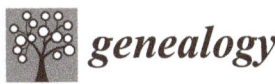

Book Review

Book Review: The Psychology of Family History

Pam Jarvis

Institute of Childhood and Education, Leeds Trinity University, Horsforth, Leeds LS18 5HD, UK; p.jarvis@leedstrinity.ac.uk

Abstract: This article reviews *The Psychology of Family History*. It proposes this as an excellent introductory text for ancestry research, creating a lively discussion of its effects upon individuals and potentially upon communities. The review additionally proposes that the book will be equally useful for academic and independent researchers in the relevant fields.

Keywords: family history; psychology; ancestry; identity construction

Citation: Jarvis, Pam. 2021. Book Review: The Psychology of Family History. *Genealogy* 5: 39. https://doi.org/10.3390/genealogy5020039

Received: 25 February 2021
Accepted: 11 April 2021
Published: 15 April 2021

Publisher's Note: MDPI stays neutral with regard to jurisdictional claims in published maps and institutional affiliations.

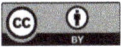

Copyright: © 2021 by the author. Licensee MDPI, Basel, Switzerland. This article is an open access article distributed under the terms and conditions of the Creative Commons Attribution (CC BY) license (https://creativecommons.org/licenses/by/4.0/).

Review

As a psychologist who is also a keen ancestry researcher, I expected to enjoy reading this book, and I was not disappointed. Moore et al. (2021) cover the growing popularity of family history/ancestry amongst the general public as well as why current populations have developed a growing interest in genealogy (slight spoiler—the advent of DNA technology forms a crucial part of this), psychological reflections on the impact of genealogical research upon the individual and ethical dilemmas which may arise in the pursuit of such research activities.

The role of religious organisations in the provision of evidence for ancestral research was also an interesting element of the book. This includes some well-considered reflections on the importance of family lineage in some religious traditions and ethical problems that some religious practices may raise—for example, that of baptising the dead.

The "who do you think you are" issue relating to the role of identity in family history research spoke personally to me as a person who started my own research with the idea that I would be principally English with two distant strands of Scottish lineage, but instead found that both paper and DNA trails showed that I was nearly half Scottish, a third continental European, and the remainder mixed Scandinavian, Irish and Kentish English. I was delighted and intrigued by this, and by the resulting reflection that my own strong nonconformist streak may have had its roots in my Scottish Covenantor and dissenting Huguenot ancestors.

However, as the writers point out, not all surprises emerging from ancestry research are positive. I have personally been aware of an incidence of a mother seeking the man who fathered her child via sperm donation through an ancestry DNA service, culminating in an emphatic message from him that he did not want his current family to be made aware of the child's existence. I have also been involved in a situation in which a woman discovered records of a still-living, unexpected half-sister of her very elderly mother's, with neither woman being aware that the other existed. In both cases, the information was not made available to those who would have been most heavily impacted by it, but through a chain of events in which others had been presented with very difficult choices about what to reveal to whom. These issues are thoroughly discussed in the text, with reference to adoption and forced adoption, with emphasis upon some characteristically Australian experiences of this issue, reflecting the authors' Australian origins.

Some of the topics covered are so new that there is little supporting research evidence to draw upon, such as ancestry research issues raised by the donation of gametes and surrogacy agreements. This sometimes caused the discussion and analysis in the text to become somewhat speculative. I also felt that the authors could have extended the analysis of ancestry research through the perspective of identity theory to reduce the heavy reliance upon Ericksonian theory (Orenstein and Lewis 2020). The context of social constructionism (Misra and Prakash 2012) would have lent an interesting angle to this analysis in terms of how we construct our personal identities in flexible ways, which are likely to be enhanced by the addition of knowledge about our unique ancestral combinations. For example, the synthesis of my own genealogical blending of a potent mixture of ancestral dissenters discussed above is a very personal take. Others with the same combination of genes might create many different narratives from the same information.

The impact upon stories that we tell about ourselves from the perspective of revealed family history would be a fascinating research topic in itself. However, as far as I am aware, it has not been covered in currently available academic publications. This takes the book to the crux of its dilemma—the newness of the popular ancestry fascination and the recency of the DNA component (Royal et al. 2010), resulting in sparsity of underpinning academic literature. As such, this led the last third of the book in particular to making a significant amount of speculative commentary, which is nevertheless interesting in itself—for example, the potential benefits and drawbacks of engagement in ancestry research.

The authors make some useful suggestions relating to the use of ancestry research in demonstrating to children that they have roots within a genetic and cultural heritage and in helping grandparents to feel that they are leaving a legacy for their descendants, and in documenting much loved relatives who have been dead for some time to permit them to "live" to some extent in the minds of their descendants.

As a family researcher who took one of her ancestral family stories into a novel, I can also relate to the drawbacks the authors suggest: the temptation to live more in the past than the present, and the overwhelming sadness created by the knowledge of some of the plights in which ancestors found themselves, particularly those that could be much more easily solved in the present, which is one of the key themes of the novel in question.

The authors make some salient suggestions for the use of ancestry research in therapy for grief and raise the possibility that ancestry research may usefully cross the family/formal history research barrier as a pedagogic device to render people in history more relatable to schoolchildren as fellow human beings. I have personal experience of this process too, having many years ago taken in a photograph of my long dead grandfather as a child to talk to my children's primary class about Victorians. A child in the class pointed out that my grandfather looked very similar to my son "dressed up" and stated that therefore he was now convinced that Victorians must have been "real".

I would add to this that through such study, children could also discover immigrant heritage of which they were previously unaware, which could be used as a thinking tool to reduce discrimination and prejudice against more recent immigrants. For example, I experienced a powerful reflection on this point when I discovered that the word "refugee" passed into English through my Huguenot ancestors' language.

In summary, there is a lot to recommend this book to anyone who wants to learn a little more about ancestry research, its effects upon researchers and potentially, the wider community. Its only downfall is that, sometimes, the underpinning research is somewhat sparse, meaning that consequently, the text begins to move into a rather speculative arena. However, on the other hand, the book is written in a format that makes it an excellent candidate for the nonacademic ancestry interest market. It is an easy, absorbing read and its terminology will be easily grasped by hobbyist family researchers, who I am sure would find its contents highly interesting and informative.

Institutional Review Board Statement: Not applicable.

Informed Consent Statement: Not applicable.

Data Availability Statement: Not applicable.

Conflicts of Interest: The author declares no conflict of interest.

References

Misra, Girishwar, and Anand Prakash. 2012. Kenneth J. Gergen and Social Constructionism. *Psychological Studies* 57: 121–25. Available online: https://link.springer.com/article/10.1007/s12646-012-0151-0#citeas (accessed on 25 February 2021).

Moore, Susan, Doreen Rosenthal, and Rebecca Robinson. 2021. *The Psychology of Family History*. Abingdon: Routledge.

Orenstein, Gabriel, and Lindsay Lewis. 2020. Erickson's Stages of Psychosocial Development. In *StatPearls*. Available online: https://www.ncbi.nlm.nih.gov/books/NBK556096/ (accessed on 25 February 2021).

Royal, Charmaine D., John Novembre, Stephanie M. Fullerton, David B. Goldstein, Jeffrey C. Long, Michael J. Bamshad, and Andrew G. Clark. 2010. Inferring Genetic Ancestry: Opportunities, Challenges, and Implications. *American Journal of Human Genetics* 86: 661–73. Available online: https://www.ncbi.nlm.nih.gov/pmc/articles/PMC2869013/ (accessed on 25 February 2021).

MDPI
St. Alban-Anlage 66
4052 Basel
Switzerland
Tel. +41 61 683 77 34
Fax +41 61 302 89 18
www.mdpi.com

Genealogy Editorial Office
E-mail: genealogy@mdpi.com
www.mdpi.com/journal/genealogy

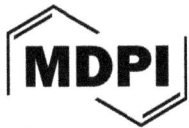

www.ingramcontent.com/pod-product-compliance
Lightning Source LLC
LaVergne TN
LVHW070617100526
838202LV00012B/666